THE HEALER'S WAY

Praise for Rahul Patel's *The Healer's Way**

Rahul Patel's transformational pathway is a guide that many can follow. Fascinating reading.

> – Louise L. Hay, author of *You Can Heal Your Life*

Rahul Patel has that rare ability to motivate people to change, which is a vital quality possessed by great healers.

> – Larry Dossey, M.D., author of *Healing Words: The Power of Prayer and the Practice of Medicine.*

Rahul Patel has a very complete understanding of the role of the mind-body connection in illness and in health. He is very effective in demonstrating the impact of joy and zest for life in the healing process.

> – O. Carl Simonton, M.D., author of *Getting Well Again*

I am hearing more and more about your extraordinary ability to open people's hearts, inspiring them with your eclectic and authoritative knowledge of Energy Medicine.

> – Candace Pert, Ph.D., author of *Molecules of Emotion: The Science Behind Mind-Body Medicine*

Rahul is a unique and gifted being. As one of today's most amazing and humbling healers, he delves into the language of the soul and demonstrates the potential of the human heart.

> – James Van Praagh, author of *Talking to Heaven: A Medium's Message of Life After Death*

Rahul Patel: his work and book are informative and exciting. Exposure to the man and his work is a healing experience.

> – Bernie Siegel, M.D., author of *Love, Medicine and Miracles*

* *Endorsements collected in preparation for the publication of the work in 2003.*

THE HEALER'S WAY

An Inner Guide to Healing Through ENERGY MEDICINE

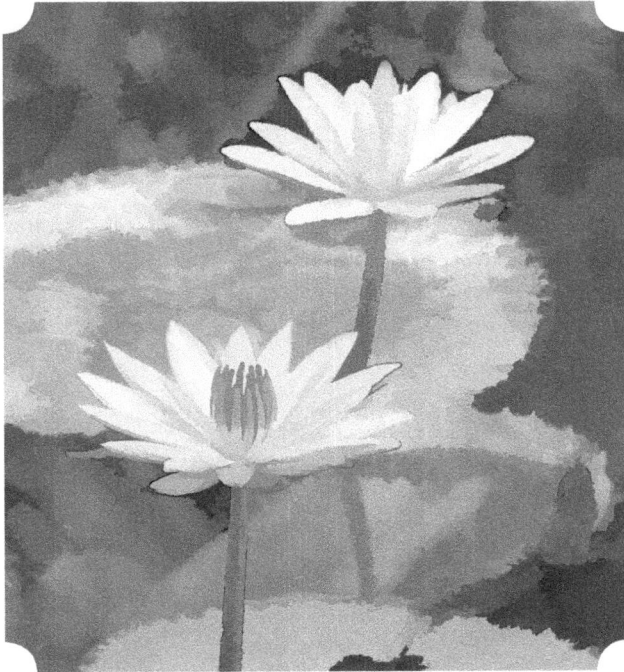

RAHUL PATEL

With forward by Neale Donald Walsch

Cover photo and interior photo of Rahul Patel
provided by Dorothy Seeger

ISBN 978-1-952194-05-4

Design by River Sanctuary Graphic Arts

Printed in the United States of America

The author, editor and publisher make no claim of any kind regarding the methods included in this book. It is recommended to always consult with your physician. These methods for healing and health are to be used at the reader's discretion.

Additional copies available from:

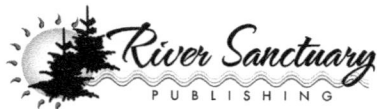

www.riversanctuarypublishing.com

amazon.com

River Sanctuary Publishing
P.O Box 1561
Felton, CA 95018
www.riversanctuarypublishing.com

Dedicated to the awakening of the New Earth

*To God, my Friend, the greatest physician of all,
without Whose constant presence and limitless
miracles this book would not have been possible.*

*To my parents, whose duaah brought me back to life,
to whom I am forever grateful.*

To the Bird who is still flying.

The Birds sing, not because they have answers,
They sing because they have songs.

The Healer's Way is a journey of finding
the *Song of Life*

R A H U L   P A T E L

CONTENTS

Contents, cont.

PART THREE — HEALING THE SPIRIT

❀

FOREWORD

From the beginning of time, human beings have been trying to find the secret of healing the diseases which rack our bodies. We've invented medicines and procedures, created buildings and marvelous machines, and, in all, done a pretty good job in some areas – although not nearly as good a job as we might have done with none of this…

The truth is, we have within us the power to heal any condition. The problem is, not very many people believe that. Many people want to believe that, but not very many people do. That is because we live in a world which is conditioned, and indeed created, by our previous thoughts on a subject and by the environment and the reality which those prior thoughts have produced.

We have thought for a long time that healing the body with energy which we can control with our minds is impossible and so, of course, it is. Unless, of course, you are one of those who hold a different thought about it.

The problem is compounded by the fact (I am sorry to say) that very powerful elements in our world have a huge vested interest in all of us continuing our disbelief in the power of energy as medicine. There is no need here to get into who or what those powerful elements are. Books have already been written on that subject. What is important is to simply acknowledge that there are people in high places who do not want us to know that, when it comes to health and healing, there is another way.

Yet not all of the "established order" is in denial, and more and more we are seeing breakdowns of traditional systems of thought on this subject, and breakthroughs which, even a few years ago, we might not have imagined. The Associated Press sent a startling article across its wires not long ago headlined *Medical Students Take Course On Spirituality:*

"Medical students expect to study the hard sciences. To help make them better doctors, Wake Forest University is also asking them to take on something more ethereal – religion.

"'It's as important as good nutrition and exercise,' said S. Bryant Kendrick Jr., an ordained minister who is also on the faculty of Wake Forest's Bowman Gary School of Medicine. 'Contemplative Meditation is like a good drug,' he said. 'The body was made for prayer.'

"Kendrick said the grant is further proof of the recognition within the medical community that spirituality has an important role in the overall health care of patients.

"Evidence is growing that religion can be good medicine. At the annual meeting of the American Association for the Advancement of Science earlier this year, researchers who reviewed 212 studies said they found three-fourths showed a positive effect of religious commitment on health.

"The medical School in Winston-Salem was one of six in the country to receive a $10,000 John Templeton Foundation grant. The award is to be used to teach medical students how to incorporate spirituality into clinical care." (reprinted with the permission of the Associated Press.)

Now, isn't that interesting? Yet we don't have to await the results of this "new" experiment. We already know the truth about all this. We have been told over and over again through the centuries, and by such notable recent teachers as Deepak Chopra, Wayne Dyer, Bernie Siegel and Elisabeth Kübler-Ross.

Now comes another wonderful teacher, Rahul Patel, with a first-hand account that solidifies our understanding, and makes it real. This is a wonderful, gentle, easy-to-read "how to" book that may be used to great benefit. It de-mystifies the mystifying, and as such is a wonderful gift.

Conversations with God says that we create our own reality with three Tools of Creation: Thought, Word and Deed. It also says that our health is a reflection of our state of mind, and that human beings were meant to live very, very much longer than they now do.

The Healer's Way, not surprisingly, says the same thing – and further, describes *how*. Offered by a man who himself has "cheated death," this volume contains down-to-earth, practical advice on healing the mind, body and spirit. This book is perfect for those who doubt and for those who have never doubted, but also have never been given specific ways to put their faith into action. Use what Rahul Patel here calls "Energy Medicine" and no matter how long you live, your life will be more peaceful, more serene, and healthier in every way.

Neale Donald Walsch, author
Conversations with God

🏵 PREFACE

"I want you to publish my book," said Rahul Patel to me in August of 2004, shortly after I became his assistant. "It tells about my path to becoming a healer. There should be no changes made and I want it published by a major publishing house, not independently published." He emphasized particularly that nothing should be changed.

It seemed a tall order – to find a publisher who would not only accept the book, but would agree not to make any changes. Fortunately for me at that time, Mr. Patel did not give me the manuscript and I was not required to undertake what, to me, seemed like an impossible task, even though the Forward was written by Neale Donald Walsh.

The manuscript for *The Healer's Way* rested quietly where Rahul Patel had put it until after he left his body in February of 2012 when his brother, Ambarish Patel, who had come from India, went through Rahul's belongings. He found the manuscript, 200 unbound pages printed on one side, and, not wanting to get involved with publishing, left it with me. However, since he is the legal owner of the book and did not assign any rights to me, I could not legally publish it.

There was another long wait until December of 2019 when a former student of Mr. Patel offered to copy the manuscript and have it spiral bound. For the first time I was able to read the whole book. It brought up memories of the 9-volume CD set by Rahul Patel, *Energy Healing*, which was published by Nightingale-Conant, a leading audio publisher of spiritual authors. Mr. Patel told me once that he had spoken the whole set at one sitting without stopping and the lady who was recording it was in tears when he finished. In his introduction, Mr. Patel indicates that his book was written the same way, as a torrent of wisdom.

Although Mr. Patel finished the book in 1999, it is still inspiring and useful for those seeking a healing way of life. I felt it should be published as Mr. Patel wished. I wrote by email to Ambarish Patel and told him of my wish to publish independently, hoping that as the legal owner, he would give his blessing to the effort. I received no reply, so I assumed that he had no objection to my publishing this compendium of healing wisdom.

I am very grateful to Violeta Cu Unjieng for her assistance and to Annie Elizabeth Porter of River Sanctuary Publishing in Felton, California, for her guidance in turning the manuscript into a book.

It is my wish that *The Healer's Way* will fulfill Rahul Patel's dream, honor his life and teachings, and spark a current of energy for both healers and those seeking healing.

Dorothy Seeger, editor
Oakland, California
June 2020

INTRODUCTION

Life is a continuum of energy. We live in this continuum. Like the fish who swims in the ocean, yet knows it not, we live in a boundless ocean of energy, unaware of its full potential. All that is required is our consciousness. Energy creates our three-dimensional world, our hologram of possibilities. The dimensions of our hologram are Mind, Body and Spirit. Mind creates logic, Body creates harmony and Spirit creates magic. We are living celebrations of energy.

When I wrote this book, this book was actually writing me. I channeled through consciousness that tells me that God is not in heaven but is personified in each one of us if we are willing to receive. The word Kabbala, comes from qibbel, meaning to receive. This book is the result of my receiving messages from Spirit – that life is a magical symphony when we find our path. The messages are always there if we but step aside and let them come through.

We have evolved from warriors to lovers. The way of the warrior predominated in prehistoric times. The warrior was king, and power was his instrument. Force was the weapon, and will was the motive. The way of the lover grew out of matriarchal influences as man acknowledged the amazing power of woman to give birth to new life. This awareness celebrated the goddess energies. The heart was the center of the lover's way. Surrender was the secret.

The warrior and the lover are both incomplete without the interplay of one another. There is an eternal dance between the god and the goddess, the animus and the anima, the cosmic aspects of male and female principles contained within each of us.

The Healer's Way is the merging of these complementary energies. As we are going into the new millennium, I believe we are entering an age of the healers. We can clone many things, but we can not clone consciousness. I invite you to unfurl the spinnaker of your heart and join me on a journey, The Healer's Way, the way of Energy Medicine.

Our mind is digital, and our faith is analog. A digital approach is newly-evolved and mechanistic. An analog approach is primordial and integrated. Healing primarily occurs in our analog system. Medical professionals tend to be digital, and ignore the holistic nature of the organism, choosing to cure rather than to heal. In healing we enter into the basic imprint of existence, the hologram of our possibilities. We heal the dichotomy between digital and analog, male and female, will and surrender.

The Greek philosopher and poet, Empedocles, said "God is a circle whose center is everywhere, and its circumference is nowhere." In our playful consciousness we find that center which Krishna described as Leela – divine play. I was searching for ways to heal with energy. I went to China, Tibet, Japan Africa and Egypt to discover and experience healing with energy. The basic thing I learned was, that by finding the center within, we heal. That center is known by different names in different cultures. That center is the hub of Energy Medicine. The beauty of Energy Medicine is that it is available here-and-now, and no insurance plan is required. We do not have to go anywhere to buy it or find it. We are the sole creators of Energy Medicine.

This book is about discovery, about finding ways to wholeness. There is no "later" in the realm of healing, all we have is the eternal now. As long as there is a spark of hope in our hearts, we can summon the energy to heal anything. We can journey from loss to abundance. We can journey from hurt to love. We can journey from wounded-ness to wholeness. When there is darkness, we do not remove it. We bring light – the light of love, the light of hope, the light of Oneness. All light reflects from the same source, Spirit.

Energy is a flow. Nothing dies in the world of energy. Spirit is our innate potential, our connection with divinity. God is energy, that is why energy can heal. Matter in high energy physics does not die but undergoes a process of transmutation; form changes. In the world of energy, we undergo transformation; we change. As Goethe said, "that moment one definitely commits oneself, then Providence moves too…" Whatever you can do, or dream you can, begin it. Boldness has genius and power and magic in it…

We heal ourselves by giving the very thing we desire. We become whole by transforming from passion to compassion. Passion is our individual flame of creativity. Compassion is sharing that flame with others. Honoring the Spirit in everyday life is celebrating the sacred. Sacredness gives meaning and purpose to our ordinary lives.

Spirit is the ecosystem of our existence. In the world of Spirit, we transcend. In the realm of Energy Medicine, we transform. It is a journey we take from the self to the Spirit when we open our hearts. Our consciousness leads us to joy, and joy leads us along our path. Where there is joy, there is healing.

This is a book of transformation. Welcome to the path. As we walk together, if I have touched a heart, a soul, a person, I feel the energy has connected us.

Pranaam,

Rahul Patel, California
Twice in a blue moon, March 31, 1999

The Healer's Way: An Inner Guide to Healing Through Energy Medicine is a sacred offering that sings the glory of Spirit. As there are many people, there are many paths; there is no one way to God's garden. The fuel of energy is Spirit. By personally connecting to Spirit, we begin our healer's journey. I believe that all healing comes from that Spirit, but we have to mobilize the innate power we all have, our gift from God. This innate power lies dormant in all of us. In a crisis or in a call of Spirit, the inner alchemy of transformation can begin. We don't have to wait for a crisis. We can start today .

The Healer's Way is a path of compassion. When we love ourselves the way we are, we begin our journey, where energy becomes the medicine of healing. The right to live comes from the rites of Spirit!

Rahul Patel

PART ONE

Healing the Mind

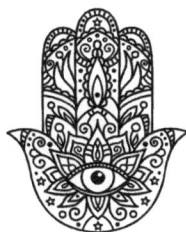

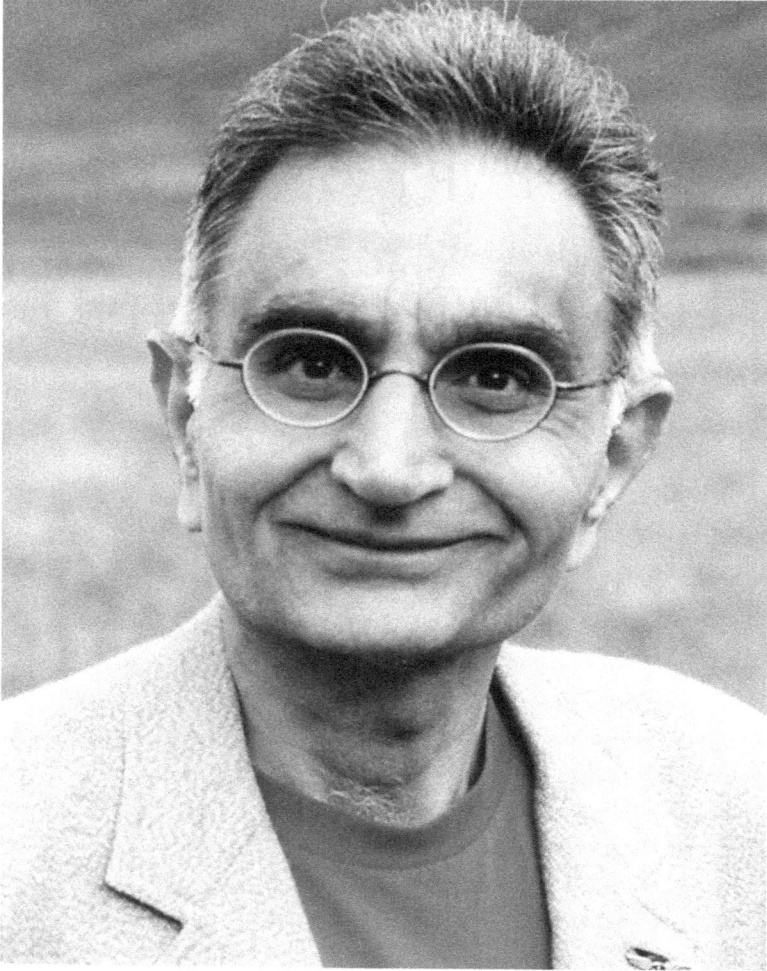

Rahul "Star" Patel

✾

CHAPTER I

THE HEALER'S JOURNEY

My Own Story

One has to harbor in chaos in order to
give birth to your Dancing Star.

— *Nietzsche*

Writing this book is, for me, like offering a prayer in the most difficult hour, like lighting a candle in the dark – to bring luminosity and light.

Life is dynamic. Change is our only certainty. It is the hub of Natural Law around which all else revolves. The sun, moon, tides, and all of life, remain in perpetual motion, and at each moment are born anew. Change provides our vital essence. It is the only constant on which we can depend. This book is part of the same dynamic law, and everything that you are going to read will change.

I never imagined that my life would actually begin when my world collapsed. More than twelve years ago, doctors told me that I had only a few months to live because I had been diagnosed with lung cancer.[1] I felt as if I had received my death sentence.

I was living in the United States at that time and I decided to go to England to explore new options for healing. The British tend to adopt a minimalist approach in medicine, *do less of nearly everything*, according to Lynn Payer, renowned author of the book *Medicine and Culture*.[2] This orientation is based on the classical Hippocratic "do no harm" dictum that encourages and supports the body's own natural healing processes. I had always believed that nature provides us with

3

intelligence, from the innate intelligence locked within our DNA to the natural rhythms inherent within all life. The "secrets" are only secrets until we learn to listen to nature. We are better off honoring the Tao[3] of life.

I went to an expert pulmonologist in London, who served as my primary physician. We discussed my options. He recommended that I undergo a stat CT scan to explore a massive area of scarring in my lungs that was located close to my heart.

Having no acquaintances in the Western world, I went to India and brought the strength of my family back with me. I believed that a sense of connection was essential to my well-being. My mother, father, brother and uncle flew to London, the Land Where the Sun Never Sets, a place to find the Light.

The same day the surgeon was going to perform my lung biopsy, a motorbike-messenger arrived with my latest CT scan results. My primary pulmonologist interpreted these results for me in his consultation room. He reported that there was good news and bad news. The good news, "You don't need lung surgery." The bad news, "You have a tumor the size of an orange in your kidney." He added, "No one can expect to live for long with a tumor of that size untreated. It is remarkable that you are still alive."

The doctor immediately called one of the premier urological surgeons in Europe with consent from me and my family. Fortunately, this surgeon was in England at that time. He agreed to perform the operation early the following week.

Unable to afford cab fare, my family and I headed to the subway on foot to meet the surgeon. My mind was exploding with a thousand questions, and my universe was spinning. En route to the South Kensington station, my father, mother and l found a green bench, and rested as a Trinity.[4]

l was amazed. Sitting there, I became aware of a fascinating paradox; l was directly experiencing the process of destruction and creation simultaneously at that very moment. On the one hand, my life was being threatened. On the other hand, creative forces were being activated by my father's words. I distinctively remember him saying to me, "I will give you my kidney." He put his arm around me, and the three of us cried on that green bench, holding each other, overcome by gratitude.

Instantly, something profoundly changed. What was happening on the bench was that I had two conflicting "voices" inside of me. One voice was saying, "I am finished, so I do not want to live" while the other was shouting defiantly, "I want to live, and I will find my way." A light went on. I was completely flooded with hope. At that moment, I decided to live. I decided to do anything and everything to live. There was only the one voice inside me now, the voice of life. That green bench on Brampton Hospital Road became a sacred place of pilgrimage for me, which I visit frequently.

According to Newsweek (November 28, 1994 edition), a majority of Americans (58%) report they feel the need to experience spiritual growth; they are motivated to strive for something more. 45% surveyed have experienced a sense of sacredness outside of structured religion. That is exactly what I was experiencing at that holy moment. Even today, that bench is a seat of power for me.

Joseph Campbell addressed the intimate relationship between power and myth. To Campbell, mythology represented the melody of the cosmos. Today we demonstrate little interest in the ancient mysteries that serve as a loom linking all of humankind, both past and present, in an ageless weaving. In our modern preoccupation with mechanistic thought and pursuits, we have, in a sense, severed ourselves from the roots of our own family tree. We live in a society that is alienated from sacred myth. This estrangement is the genesis of our contemporary and ubiquitous breakdown, as society fragments into individuals isolated from the Oneness.

Unless and until we develop an intimate connection with some object that becomes a special symbol of power in our everyday lives, we cannot begin our healing journeys. Mythological symbols and stories are omnipresent and deeply rooted in our everyday lives, but we must look for them.

We need a daily living **mandala**.[6] A mandala need not be a circle. When we make a personal connection with any object, it becomes a healing mandala. Our personal mandalas can be anything our heart desires – a pet, a rock, a feather, a picture, a boat, a letter, even a word in a book, or a bench.

In England, the surgeon is addressed as "Mister." After reviewing all my medical test results, Mr. Grant Williams said, "I have to remove your entire kidney. This is major surgery, and I cannot give you any guarantees about the outcome, whether you will live or not. If I were you, I'd go out and have a lovely dinner." It struck me that it may be my last supper. But something happened to me. I wondered, *Is life a divine comedy?* At that critical moment, I learned to laugh. I realized that joy could be found in life's bleakest moments. Ironically, Mr. Williams' humor was a lifeline for me.[7]

He then told us the cost of the operation. A seemingly interminable silence followed as we struggled to digest the news. While whispering among ourselves, my mother spoke out and said, "Yes. We will pay." She spoke with poise, "We will sell my jewelry, use your father's savings, and you will have the necessary surgery." In honor of the hope my mother generated, the first initial of her name – "S" – remains a personal mandala for me to this day. I also persuaded the surgeon to allow my mother to stay in the hospital with me.

In an operating room overlooking the Thames River, a team of doctors performed the day-long surgery. My entire family waited anxiously outside in a prayerful state. Prayer also was initiated in several other places.[8]

After surgery, I then was transported by gurney back to my room. Shortly thereafter, I underwent another medical crisis. If not for my parents, I would not be alive today. My mother saw blood pouring through the tubes onto the rug beside my bed, and called for emergency medical assistance. A second time that day I was brought unconscious to the same operating theater, this time with tremendous blood loss. They found matching blood for a transfusion, and the team conducted a second operation.

Twice that day I died. I had lost all vital signs on two separate occasions. It was a miracle that I came back.

I saw lights… then I saw a blank. I heard the silence… I felt the Void… and I slipped into the void in silence.[9] And in that silence, someone was with me. A Voice. A Light. A Person. I was not alone. I was with God. All along, I felt as weightless as a feather, and as expansive as the wind. I was able to observe the whole experience around me in its entirety. This experience liberated me. I felt a sense of freedom I had never felt before… I came back.

When I opened my eyes, I was in my room with my family in the cold midnight of early winter. They were all surrounding me and touching me with tenderness, and saying something to me that I don't remember. But I do remember the clear "message" that I was receiving:

To live – give.

The Voice also was saying, "You have the energy within you and around you, but you must be willing to walk the path. I give you life that you will carry forth the potential of this Energy for healing."

The realization that came to me at that moment was that all life stems from the One Source. It was a reminder to return to that center of all creation. The path to that Source is through sound medicine, healing foods, laughter and celebrating all the senses within my own vibrations.[10] This brings liberation from a painful past. I must connect with the Source and share that healing with all. This is the alpha and the omega of Energy Medicine.[11]

Death brings transformation from one way of understanding to a deeper and broader view of Life. It brings clarity from chaos. It is a gift of transcendence that enables us to let go of old concepts and beliefs rooted in separation that cause pain and fear. My friend Dannion Brinkley, author of *Saved by the Light*, chronicled his own experience of looking ahead into the darkness. Brinkley described the tunnel coming to him, as he effortlessly sped toward the light where he experienced ineffable nonjudgmental compassion and love.

I experienced this unconditional love. I suddenly was bathed in gratitude. Grudges that I had harbored for eons against my father, my mother, my uncle and my brother melted away in a millisecond. For the first time in my life, my heart joined with their hearts. This heart-to-heart healing has become the cornerstone of my work. I have never slept one night since then without the ritual of saying "thank you" in several languages. I also ask for mutual forgiveness and release from any person I might have struggled with during that day.[12]

The disease that I was diagnosed with was severe, and I knew that I had to have greater faith than that disease. Faith, which brings hope, became my realization and an essential link in the Healer's Journey.

It is not something outside ourselves that we do that heals. It is our **belief** in what we do that heals. Action without faith is not healing. My faith enabled me to walk barefoot on fire several times in Santa Fe, New Mexico, several years later. When a bleeding woman was healed by touching the hem of his garment, Jesus said:

Thy faith hath made thee whole.[13]

Another discovery came to me along my Healer's Journey. I had to have a tremendous will to walk through this uncharted land of mystery but I also was privileged to gain new insights into the power of surrender.[14]

Before our departure, my surgeon reported that the excised kidney was confirmed to be malignant. He advised complete bed-rest, recommending that I return to India with my family. "There's no substitute for family," Mr. Williams emphasized.

I refused to use a wheelchair, although it was recommended. Accessing some type of extra-human strength, I extended my right foot and began to walk the day after my kidney was removed. This was a turning point. This was where the Healer's Journey began.

My return to India was booked through the busiest hub in the world, London's Heathrow International Airport. Despite the urgings of well-meaning doctors and skycaps, I once again refused a wheelchair, stubbornly insisting on making my way through the crowd without assistance. I was walking forward with a sea of humanity swirling around me, propelled by my own volition. Consciously and unconsciously, I knew my body would cooperate if I was unwavering in following my instincts. The journey of a thousand miles begins with a single step.[15]

Later, my colleague and friend, Bernie Siegel, M.D., also discovered that rapid healing often happened to those difficult and demanding patients who do not always acquiesce to the wishes of their doctors. Dr. Siegel prescribes creative ways for patients to stand up for themselves. For example, if a patient feels that they have been given a "number" rather than a name, he encourages them to be equipped with a water-gun and blow horn to be utilized when they feel mistreated while in the hospital. In order to heal, Dr. Siegel says the patient has to become a person by becoming empowered and playful.[16] It is up to the patient to create their own reality, which often may require refusing the verdict of the physician.[17]

In her authoritative research book *The Type C Connection: The Behavioral Links to Cancer and Your Health*, Lydia Temoshok, Ph.D.,[18] describes the Type C individual as being appeasing and unfailingly pleasant. Moreover, Type C persons may have an increased risk of developing cancer and have poorer outcomes in recovery. On our arrival back in India, my younger brother came to receive us with the traditional welcome of garlands. He placed a garland around each of our necks. I was speechless. My tears spoke for me. He drove us to Agra, the city of the Taj Mahal, where my family lived. I was grateful yet I felt that I could not give my parents and family what they gave me, the gift of life born anew.

After a few days had passed, many relatives began calling to inquire about the status of my health. I did not like this because it was a constant reference to the painful past. I was lying in bed, encircled in eight pillows. My father was counseling me to start a new life in India, where I had the support of family and friends. Something inside of me was telling me to move on. I decided to follow my intuition, against everyone's advice, to find my "home." I trusted my intuition, and went against the drift.

Jesus teaches about the healing of a blind man in Bethsaida. A blind man was brought to Jesus, and he was healed. And then Jesus said:

Send him home. Do not go into the village.[19]

I knew in my heart that I was searching for home. I was leaving my village, India, where I was born and raised. I was seeking a true homecoming, transcending a sense of tribal consciousness.[20] Home is not only found on the outside. It also can be found within.

On the journey to finding my home, I returned to meet with Mr. Williams to check out what he had to say regarding my follow-up. After seeing me, he was conflicted about whether or not chemotherapy was indicated. He sent me to a top-notch oncologist in another hospital for a second opinion.

The white-coated oncologist strongly recommended that I undergo chemotherapy and in mid-sentence, I interrupted him asking, "With my condition, having one kidney and a fist full of determination, has anybody ever lived with lung cancer?" He replied, "I don't know." I told him to write the following in my medical chart: "I am going to live a full life span without your treatment, and I am going to show you." And I walked out.

I was drawn to the West – I wished to return to America. I felt that many people there were of a highly evolved consciousness; that is, they were aware of their spiritual identities in a materialistic world. I felt at home with them. Something inside told me specifically to move to Los Angeles because it was called the City of Angels.

After arriving in Los Angeles, and not knowing what to do next, I started going to nearby Lafayette Park. I felt happy to see the trees, and to see people playing. I approached some older people who were standing in the sun. I had never seen them before but I was guided by a Light. I began talking without any motives. We were all smiling, and a warm sense of familiarity embraced us. I felt better. I felt stronger. I realized that the vitality surging within me was actually generated by **psychic induction**, a form of force coming from them to me and vice-versa. This exchange of energy produces heightened vibrations and increases the flow of energy that helps us to connect easily with others.[21]

When we give something from the heart, and create a true heart-to-heart connection, we induce energy. We induce life. At any time we are feeling lost, we can use psychic induction and we will experience a rejuvenating surge. I uncovered this as a significant link in the Healer's Journey. I always use psychic induction in approaching "strangers" anywhere – in malls, theaters, grocery stores bus stops, banks, and airports – indeed, everywhere! By practicing psychic induction we gain wings.

In Marilyn Ferguson's landmark book *The Aquarian Conspiracy* I learned about a doctor named Carl Simonton, a radiation oncologist. Dr. Simonton left traditional practice in favor of treating cancer patients with visualization techniques. I also discovered that he was based in Los Angeles. I then traveled 1-1/2 hours via bus to Pacific Pallisades to meet Dr. Simonton, co-author of the best-selling book *Getting Well Again*. Initially, he was not able to see me because he was busy. The second time I went, I met with Dr. Simonton. I shared my story with him. He looked at my x-rays and we talked about my journey. I told him how much impact his writing and his method had had on me, how it had amazed me to find that through visualization, we can heal one of the most dreaded of diseases.

He saw the extraordinary recovery that I had been through. He looked in my eyes and told me that I had to share my experience of healing, that it would be of great benefit for people to hear about such an experience from someone with first hand knowledge. He invited me to teach a group of cancer patients that he was treating.

I started by presenting aromatherapy, a technique that can help patients change their past memories. Later, as my evening session progressed, a few patients asked me to lay my hands on them, which I did. One of the patients, a bald physician, asked me to lay my hands on his head where his brain tumor was, and he started sobbing. I embraced him compassionately.

Next to me a middle-aged man was telling me to place my hand on his wife's chest (I later learned she was suffering from breast cancer). A few days later, I received a hand-written note from Michigan. To my surprise, this gentleman wrote that his wife's tumor had disappeared. He signed-off fondly, "Your two fans from Michigan."

I was praying in the morning, when suddenly the Voice spoke to me. I listened:

Now you have the gift of laying on hands.[22]

From then on I started placing both of my hands on my lungs every day after prayer to heal. When my next routine X-ray was done, to my surprise, the largest scar that was to be biopsied next to my heart was completely gone. It had totally disappeared. I experienced the miraculous power of my own healing touch.

Often I used to bleed profusely from my mouth. Since I had no insurance and no place to go, I devised a way that, every time that happened, I would yield to the earth, and kneel down. I then would place both hands, in faith, near my chest. Eventually, after 20-30 minutes, the bleeding would stop. I witnessed the power of my gift of laying on of hands in some of my darkest hours.

It appeared I imbibed some mystical powers that propelled me forward on my Healer's Journey. It seemed like the **magical passes**, shamanistic techniques for evolving our consciousness, on which Carlos Castañeda's Tensegrity is based.[23] Magical passes help redistribute the energy as a means of becoming conscious of the cohesive force which is in and around us. By being aware of and directing this force, we can facilitate energy healing.

To continue on the path of giving, I started going to a Jewish convalescent center, which I continue to do today. I went to cheer up the elderly patients, to bring them water and to bring provisions as needed, but mostly to give them energy and emotional support. I began to notice that many good things were happening to me. It seemed that, effortlessly, I was receiving many blessings.

I went and sat quietly and a vision came to me that I would be teaching from then on and healing with energy.

I wrote and sent this vision to the organizers of a holistic health conference in Pasadena. They responded with their interest, and I soon received an invitation to speak. At that same conference, many notables such as Dr. Elisabeth Kubler-Ross and Dr. Deepak Chopra spoke also. Although I had never spoken publicly before, I was suddenly in a venue where many people heard my words.

I continued in this work, and a number of people at conferences where I was presenting began coming to me for hands-on-healing, even though I never advertised about these gifts being available. I also started receiving numerous requests for distance healing by the power of prayer, and their number continues to grow today.

In a national conference in Santa Monica, California, I met Dr. Bernie Siegel, whose book *Love, Medicine and Miracles* I had read in 1987 after my surgery. He heard my story, and he took an angel pin from his lapel and placed it on my jacket. He said, "You are my hero." To this day that angel pin remains a mandala on my home altar, along with a picture of me with Dr. Siegel.

Bernie suggested that conference participants become bus conductors and hand out cookies to the people because he said *he had never seen so many miserable people in one place* (as on public transit). Instead of becoming a bus conductor, I became a flower boy. I started working in a floral shop during the mornings.[24] In the afternoons, I helped to heal others, and my evenings were spent researching, reading and praying.

The big blessings are Abundance. A custom-made position was created for me to work as a healing consultant in a health food store. There a major television station interviewed me and pondered, "We've heard of nutritional consultants and weight-loss experts, but we've never heard of a healing consultant!"

A group of gentlemen approached me about locating some type of health-related product in the store. One of them has become an angel of abundance for me. That was Milton Katselas, the world-renowned film director, teacher and artist. He talks about *abbondanza*, abundance. He personally taught me that:

God has, yes, He has... but we have to take.

In his best-selling book, *Dreams into Action: Getting What You Want*, Milton purports that the perception of scarcity is a lie. There is more than enough of everything if we are willing to look at abundance and not at scarcity. More importantly, we must be willing to receive.

From that store, by living out these ideas of abundance, I have been transported and have traveled half of the cherished world with my friend, Milton, to whom I am thankful. I participated in a world of healing as I continued my journey.

No experience has taught me more about surrender than my sojourn to the Great Pyramid of Giza. When the Healer's Journey took me through the Queen's Chamber, the first chamber in the Pyramid, I felt as though I was suffocating. I laid down and surrendered and asked for permission, in that electromagnetic vibration, to be granted the strength to pass on into the third and final chamber, the King's Chamber.

I went through the tunnel. It reminded me of the Bardo that I experienced while in the British hospital.

I died and came back because I could surrender.

The first thing I did in the King's Chamber was to lie down without my shirt on so that my body could touch the timeless soil. My eyes closed... and I surrendered to the same void I had entered before... and suddenly I was liberated in yet another way. I was free from the time-space limitations of my mind.

After I came back I dowsed the chamber using L-shaped rods.[25] By this process, I discovered the location where the head and the foot of the Pharaoh's body had been placed for mummification prior to being placed in the sarcophagus.

I also had an instrument called an electromagnetic EM field meter.[26] This was a rare opportunity to study the electromagnetic vibrations inside the Great Pyramid. I was shocked to discover that the needle did not move. I thought that perhaps the meter had been damaged in my travels. But the truth was the magnetic field in the King's Chamber was near zero. There were no fluctuations. It was totally stable.[27]

The healing vibrations created by the geomagnetic force field caused me to feel as though time stood still. I felt like I was in the earth's womb. The near-zero electromagnetic field that I measured created the vibration to enhance my personal healing process. I later learned that lower nonfluctuating DC fields are conducive to health. High-frequency, man-made electromagnetic AC fields are related to disruptions in health.

Apart from the ability to dowse, I also realized that I had another gift, **psychic profile**. Before I could meet or talk to anybody, a psychic scan of that person would appear before me. Although at times my perception of this psychic profile was incorrect, I still received vivid pictures with striking consistency. In my healing practice, I utilize this ability of psychic profiling to "pre-view" the person I am working with, incorporating this practice with hands-on-healing.

A few years later, after the amazing experience of surrendering inside the Great Pyramid, I was drawn to the mystical land of Tibet. Tibet is the pinnacle of the golden Shangri-la, which I had dreamed of as a child. I always felt an affinity with the images I had seen of the snow covered peaks reaching into the clouds and the saffron-robed lamas. These harmonious visions seemed naturally healing to me.

The first day proved to be an adventurous journey through the land and across the Yalutsanbu River. My friend, Milton, and I obtained a permit to enter the most ancient Tibetan monastery, Samya, built in honor of the eighth-century master, Padmasambhava. The legend says that he was born from within a lotus on a lake in India. Before he came to Tibet, the people followed a pagan tradition called Bon. Using his shamanistic powers, he cleansed the land from evil spirits. It is said that Padmasambhava hid many **termas** that will eventually be uncovered by a suitable discoverer. Termas are hidden treasures or concealed teachings.[28] We can find termas anywhere in the world in countless forms.

This monastery was a majestic, three-story-high edifice full of treasures. The first floor was Tibetan, the middle floor was Chinese, and the top floor was Indian. The lama, the holy priest of the monastery, saw something in us. He took us through all three chambers to the top, to the Indian chamber, where he performed a ceremony and blessed me with the Holy Ancient Scriptures and **chiloo**.[29] Chiloo is the most sacred and cherished initiation offered by a lama.

The next day I ventured off to find the Cave of Padmasambhava where historians say he performed the sacred spiritual rites. I passed the monastery, and started climbing a series of mountains that towered more than 11,000 feet above sea level. The air was rarefied, and I was breathless. I had two helpers and a guide. The trekking was treacherous. I could not seem to pull myself together. I put my arms around the two helpers and continued climbing. I told the guide: "If something happens to me, please send my body back to where I came from." I was determined.

I refused to drink water as a faith-offering to Padmasambhava until I entered the cave. Suddenly the clouds were rumbling and rain began to pour on my face. It was like a Divine baptism. Soon we could see the gate and we entered. There was a prayer wheel at the entrance where I sat and prayed. After that I proceeded into the main cave.

I felt the same power, the timelessness, which I had felt earlier in the British hospital. I was speechless. I sat in silence where Padmasambhava must have sat over 1200 years ago. I felt my spirit being liberated. It seemed as if I was receiving spirit transmissions from Padmasambhava, and was becoming a Tibetan, a treasure discoverer, as described in *Hidden Teachings of Tibet: An Explanation of the Terma Tradition of Tibetan Buddhism.*[30] The whole vision of my future book, *The Healer's Way,* opened up before me in a flash. Outside it was thundering while I experienced this lightening-like illumination. It was here that I transcended...

...from a passion for life to compassion for others.

When I arrived back in the United States, I was still searching for my dharma.[31] I met Louise Hay, author of *You Can Heal Your Life* and she sent me a card inspiring me to contribute to bringing healing to our planet. She wrote, "Amidst the challenges of life is the opportunity for incredible growth..." A blue card with a simple message accompanied her note:

The past is over.[32]

My life continued to change in profound ways. I walked into a conference and met the renowned and enlightened Dr. Deepak Chopra. After listening to my story, he put his arms around me and said, "You are healed." I will never forget this precious moment. He then gave me a "prescription" to listen to a tape of the tenth mandala from the *Rig-Veda,*[33] one of the oldest scriptures of India. I have listened to that tape religiously every day since that time. It has helped me to change my cellular memories, to heal my body, mind and spirit.

My healer's journey continued. I heard about a remarkable man, Ernesto Contreras, M.D., in Mexico. I went to meet him and to encounter, first-hand, his alternative ways of healing. Dr. Contreras built a church and constructed a hospital. His philosophy of healing was to treat the soul first, then the body. Coupled with noninvasive alternative medicine, Dr. Contreras treated cancer patients by playing the guitar and singing them the love song, *Cielito Lindo*. He looked in my eyes knowingly, and said to me:

Go and be the hands of God and you will heal.

So what is the **Healer's Journey?** We teach what we need to learn in order to heal. All healers begin as wounded healers. When we begin our journey of healing we imbibe the power to transform. We must give and share that power freely with others. When we share with compassion, we create a magical metamorphosis from a cocoon – cages of limitation from our past – to a butterfly, our world of possibilities.

The death of a cocoon is the birth of a butterfly. As my body died on the operating table, my mind died in the King's Chamber, and my spirit was liberated in the cave...

I found myself. I found my soul.
I found my home. I was reborn.

The healer's journey is a hero's passage. The hero never dies. The hero emerges with different forms as a warrior and as a lover. When we synthesize both, representing the god and goddess within, the healer emerges.[34]

We do not have to have dis-ease to participate in the healer's journey. We can start right now, where we are at this moment. We can give love when we are lonely... celebrate when we have no riches...when it snows, we can build a snowman. According to the sacred Indian scripture, the Bhagavad-Gita:

What is real always was, and cannot be destroyed.

नासतो वद्ियते भवो नाभावो वद्ियते सत:

nāsato vidyate bhavo nābhavo vidyate satah 2:16

EXERCISES FOR TRANSFORMATION AND HEALING

1. **Heart-to-Heart Connection:** The seat of wisdom lies in
    our heart, not in our mind. At least once a day, we can find
    someone or something to connect with in a way that transports
    us beyond our past. Even making a heart-to-heart connection
    with strangers is okay, and perhaps even more fun.

2. **The Magic of Psychic Induction:** When we feel isolated, we
    can step out and bring ourselves into a situation where there is
    a flow of people and vitality. We can surround ourselves with a
    vortex of positive energy, from dining places to divine places.
    Be willing to give and receive instantly. We will be energized.

3. **The Power of Faith:** Anything we do, do it with conviction,
    knowing that the world is actually on our side. Challenge our
    fears using Faith, not mind. Faith is the bridge to miracles. For
    example, when we are afraid of heights we can go in elevators
    with faith and a friend.

4. **Sacred Surrender:** We cannot win until we are ready to
    surrender, totally accepting our current conditions by
    recognizing that there is a purpose for everything. Letting go
    of our need to control completely on the spur of the moment
    is surrender. We can practice surrender rituals by lying down
    on the earth, or under the hands of a nurturing person. We
    can then repeat, "I Am Surrender" while breathing deeply and
    slowly.

5. **Liberation of the Spirit:** Spirit is present in everything we
    do, whether or not we can see, touch or feel it. When we do
    things with a sense of sacredness in everyday life, we magnetize
    Spirit to join us! Discover one new thing each day that we can
    consider sacred and share this with a friend.

Notes

1. This seemed nearly inconceivable to me, especially, since I had been a vegetarian committed to daily holistic and spiritual practices from birth.

2. p. 101.

3. Tao, "the Way," according to Lao Tse. Indeed, when Buddhism arrived in China from India, Confucious' classifications dominated Chinese life. Classification divides. In order to become whole, one must embrace totality. Lao Tse rejuvenated the Way of Life by emphasizing the balance between contrasts in day-to-day living, and brought back the holistic way of Life.

4. According to the Greek philosopher and mathematician Pythagoras, the number "3" represents completion. In Biblical symbology, "3" represents the Father, Son and the Holy Spirit. Pagan goddess followers discovered "3" unique forms: the Mother, the Virgin and the Crone. In India, "3" signifies the Divine Trinity: Brahma, Vishnu and Mahesh, signifying the balance between Creation and Destruction.

5. Just as Adam, the first man, gave life to Eve by contributing a part of himself, my father's offer to put his own life at risk, an act of unconditional love, awakened the sleeping healer within me, and instantly renewed my lust for life.

6. Mandala: the Sanskrit word meaning "sacred circles;" an ancient universal symbol of Healing and Transformation. Colors and shapes within the circle have meaning. Mandalas are everywhere. Create them.

7. Please refer to Chapter 7: *Amuse-ology: Healing with Laughter.*

8. Back in India, my uncle's family began performing the **haven**, a ritualistic prayer of sacred chanting that takes place in front of a holy fire. Meanwhile my younger brother, who was living in Agra, was praying with other family members, and his wife was fasting (an auspicious ritual in Indian culture).

9. According to the Tibetan Book of the Dead, composed in the 8th Century, bardo is a place or a phase of preparation for the soul's evolutionary changes in the afterworld; metaphorically, it is likened to a fish leaping forth from the stream. A grey, twilight-like light can be seen in the after death scene. This "astral light" is said to be ubiquitously distributed throughout waking life, as well, albeit it is not detectable via our physical sense of vision.

10. The healing properties of sound, food and laughter are elucidated in Parts II and III.

11. Please refer to Chapter Two: *The Rebirth of Energy Medicine: New Option Global Medicine.*

12. This ritual is an essential ingredient in Energy Medicine, elaborated in Chapter Two's *Exercises for Transformation and Healing.*

13. Mark 5:26, New Testament.

14. The concept of *surrender* will be further illustrated later in this chapter.

15. Lao Tse.

16. Before I became familiar with Dr. Siegel's work, I had instinctively refused to have a kidney biopsy, contrary to the doctor's recommendation.

17. Mr. Michio Kushi, who popularized Macrobiotics in the U.S. and internationally (refer to Chapter Four: *Food that Heals: Rejuvenating the Body*), also does not believe in biopsy as a diagnostic procedure due to the risk of spreading malignancy.

18. Dr. Temoshok is the head of the U.S. Military's Behavioral Medicine Research Program.

19. *Mark 8:26, New Testament.*

20. Carolyn Myss, Ph.D., eloquently describes tribal consciousness in her best-selling book *Why People Don't Heal and How They Can.*

21. Please refer to *Exercises for Transformation and Healing* at the end of the chapter for how to practice psychic induction.

22. See *1 Corinthians 12:4-5*, "*There are many kinds of gifts but only one Spirit. There are many different services but only one Lord,*" New Testament.

23. A 20th century mystic who was seen as a bridge to the world of the unknown by millions of spiritual seekers, especially in the 1960's.

24. Apart from teaching nationally and publishing at this time, Rahul entertained the idea of having a flower shop called Serendipity where a joyful or a broken-hearted lover, a hopeless man or a rejected woman can come for a cup of soup, buy a flower, and leave the store feeling "transformed," like *angels without wings*.

25. Dowsing is a divining art; it is a search, usually with the aid of any of a number of hand-held instruments, to discover anything you wish to find.

26. These findings, and their implications for healing, are further discussed in Chapter Six, *Earth Medicine: Biology of Environment*.

27. I believe the stable energy field is related to an absence of decay process in the Great Pyramid of Giza.

28. See *Termas* section near the end of this book.

29. The photograph of the initiation is contained on the back cover.

30. Tulku Thondup Rinpoche, author.

31. A Sanskrit word that means "purpose in life."

32. To this day, I carry this card with me in my wallet.

33. See Chapter Five, *Hear and Your Soul Shall Live: The Healing Power of Sound and Music*.

34. These metaphors are elaborated in Joseph Campbell's extensive work on mythology.

✿

CHAPTER II

THE REBIRTH OF ENERGY MEDICINE

New Options for Global Medicine

Energy is eternal delight.

—William Blake

As I traveled on the Healer's Way, I have witnessed uncountable examples of healing through energy. What I learned in my travels and experienced as pragmatic results, I am now synthesizing as the rebirth of Energy Medicine. My spirit continues to guide me along the path and propels me to share how we all can heal by Energy Medicine.

In this chapter, my objective is trifold. First, I wish to condense a brief history in time, the ancestry of Energy Medicine. I then will explain how and, more importantly, why to implement Energy Medicine as an orientation-of-choice in the new millennium approach to healing. Lastly, I will present an overview of specific methods that we can begin to practice here-and-now in daily living to realize our full potential and heal.

HISTORICAL UNDERPINNINGS OF ENERGY MEDICINE

The emergence of Energy Medicine in the new millennium is not new. Throughout eternity, humankind has experienced the power in nature at the same time as we have witnessed the calamities surrounding us. From the soil of this experience, a **Global Medicine** emerged that integrated indigenous practices and regional variations of geographic and climatic adaptations. Global Medicine is defined as a primordial healing art based on the interplay between belief systems, native knowledge of the flora and fauna, food, local dialects, sound vibrations, and regional mythologies. According to the ancient Indian text, the *Rig Veda*:

> *It is the One Sun who reflects in all the ponds.*

This universal sun symbolized the dawn of Global Medicine throughout different countries of the world. The shaman, the herbalist and the healer all practiced within the bailiwick of Global Medicine. The shaman accessed the power of nature, the herbalist brought the medicinal knowledge of plants, and the healer focused on Spirit. Global Medicine represented the synthesis of this triune approach. Guido Majno, M.D., brilliantly explained this in *The Healing Hand: Man and Wound in the Ancient World*. Global Medicine brings to life the civilizations of humankind, from India under Ashoka, Hippocrates' influence in Greece, Egypt at the time of the pharaohs, to the period of Mencius in China. In that era, energy could be felt but not measured.

Global Medicine was the root from which Energy Medicine emerged. Energy was recognized as the basic ingredient in healing in the pre-technological era. The life force is the crux of Energy Medicine.

In the new epoch, energy can be measured but it is no longer felt because of our over-reliance on technology. Our modem-day, religious adherence to mechanistic thought, coupled with a dogma that tangible, numerically-based proof is scientific, disables our capacity for intuitive and perceptive intelligence. T.S. Eliot beautifully portrays this in *Choruses From "The Rock:"*

> *Where is the wisdom we have lost in knowledge?*
> *Where is the knowledge we have lost in information?*

Energy has different names in different cultures. For example, it is called **chi** in Chinese, **gana** in Latin America, **ki** in Japan, **baraka** in Sufi, and **ruach** in Kabbalistic tradition.

In Judeo-Christian tradition, the Divine breath was the essential energy of life.[1] In the *Koran*, the word **nafas** means *the breath of Allah*, God. In the Kalahari Desert in Africa, the local inhabitant Kung people called that life energy **num**. Num energy was identified by Kalaharis to be located in the base of the spine and in the lower abdomen. In Indian yogic tradition, **kundalini** is equivalent to num. The Kung also discovered that, through dance, num can peak to its highest point. This is beautifully illustrated by the author Richard Katz in his book entitled *Boiling Energy*.

It is not surprising that in the oldest healing medicine, **Ayurveda**, the crux of energy, **prana**,[2] lies in the **nabhi**, which is located near the navel. On the subcontinent of China, this reservoir of energy was called **dantian**.[3] It is interesting to know that Qigong incorporates many practices from Indian **yoga**,[4] becoming whole. Yoga far predates Qigong in the history of healing. The purpose of both ancient traditions is to invigorate one's self with more life force, and create balance by removing blocks in energy via breathing, exercise, physical movement and meditation. In ancient Greece, the philosopher Anaximenes purported that life came from the breath, or **pneuma**. The father of modern medicine, Hippocrates, taught that life force should flow. According to Hippocrates, there are three major body fluids, namely the phlegm, bile and blood. In order to be healthy, he believed in creating a balance within the three fluids.[5]

ALCHEMY OF CONTRADICTION

Life is full of contradictions. There is a space between opposing forces where balance can be reached, and healing begins. **Alchemy** is the process of transmuting base elements into a higher form.

In the medieval tradition of alchemy, there are four stages of transformation; this process of change has both material, psychological and spiritual implications. The first stage is **calcinatio**, which means burning. The second stage is **solutio**, or melting. The third phase, **coagulatio** is the process of removing moisture. It is in the fourth stage of **sublimatio** where crystallization occurs. The end result of the four phases is a transformation characterized by the marriage of contradictory elements. The end product, or final synergy, is called **coniunctio** where a new entity emerges that represents a blending of the polarities.

Alchemy is not just converting lower metals into gold. Gold is a metaphor for the highest level of spiritual attainment. The true spirit of alchemy is the personal transformation of consciousness. In our contemporary life, we can become modern alchemists. By attracting our desired destinies through synchronicity, we can transmute ordinary experiences into golden opportunities. We become the living alchemists when we begin to let go of past traumatic cellular memories without blaming, and attract new energies and supportive, nonjudgmental people into our lives.

In the dance of opposites, science and mysticism meet at a juncture. Taoism and yogic traditions highlight the same balance among apparent opposites, as the alchemists were addressing in coniunctio earlier. The *Yoga Sutras of Patanjali* suggest:

> *The acceptance of pain is a means to purify,*
> *and complete surrender to the Divine is the*
> *key to yoga in living.*

The Genesis of Energy Medicine

I often wondered how the seemingly separate paradigms of science and mysticism fit together to form a Gestalt, an all-encompassing model for healing. Energy Medicine provided an open dynamic for integrating contradictions and bringing balance.

Energy can neither be created nor destroyed. Energy is the soul that propels us in life. We cannot burn the soul with fire nor can we wet it with water.[6] The soul never dies. It is our true Light, whenever we feel damaged or devastated...

Return to the soul and become whole.

Consciousness is a stream of energy and our awareness has the power to affect that stream of energy. In scientific experiments, it has been shown that the consciousness of the observer affects energy. When scientists were observing energy, sometimes it manifested as wave and sometimes as particle. The intention of the scientist affected the outcome. This is a clear demonstration that consciousness is a nonlocal form of energy. This energy can be experienced in the power of prayer in distance healing.[7] Energy has free will, which is available to each of us. Free will is like light that travels limitlessly and does not lose its luminosity over distance.

The Essence of Energy Medicine

When this consciousness becomes aware of itself, so to speak, it gives birth to the potential to utilize energy as medicine for any type of healing. In the world of energy, everything is vibration. The basis of Energy Medicine is to connect with creative vibrations through heightening our awareness. We are responsible for attracting life-enhancing vibrations. Life is not happening to us automatically. We are the co-creators of our destinies. Through consciousness, we attract energy around us. By attracting life-enhancing vibrations, we move toward our cherished aspirations. My basic premise is that the conscious use of intention and will manifest energy. When energy merges with consciousness, Spirit overflows, creating a powerful internal pharmacy called Energy Medicine.

The application and effect of Energy Medicine can be used collectively or individually. For example, **field consciousness**[8] occurs when two or more people believe in something profoundly, and begin to direct the flow of energy toward the collective intention. That is to say that, a large group of like-minded people can create a particular outcome. The next time we feel alone, that the world is against us, we can choose to spend time with optimistic people who believe the world is on our side. This synergy can inspire a shift. Of course, it also may be good Energy Medicine to keep those people around indefinitely.

The world consists of vibrations, although this remains poorly understood. You are energy; I am energy. Between us a new entity of energy is created that is the confluence of our collective vibrations. Our collective expectations can affect our lives. Evidence of this can be found in a study conducted by David Phillips, from the University of California, San Diego. He retrospectively studied data from California death certificates spanning a 24-year period (1960-1984). Among Chinese-American senior women, their death rate was shown to be 35% lower in the week preceding the Festival of the Harvest Moon where elder women are respected.

DNA HEALING

In my own experiments on energy communications with California-based scientist Cleve Backster, I discovered that when he removed leukocyte cells from my mouth and hooked them up 15-feet away by electrodes, my thoughts instantaneously affected the removed cells. At the time I was sitting in meditation while a recording was being made by a polygraph. The moment I had a thought to ask Backster a question, before I said anything, he asked me, "What are you thinking? What is going on?"

I asked him, "How did you know?," since I had never uttered a word.

He smiled at me and said that the polygraph reading showed spike patterns at the same time my thoughts were initiated. There was an exact correlation. If cells that have been removed from the body are affected by this Energy Medicine, why can't the cells within our body be affected? This communication of Energy Medicine is the future of our healing sciences.[9]

Bio-cellular communication holds the key for healing even seemingly incurable dis-eases, like cancer and AIDS. Our bodies are miraculous compositions of over 100 trillion cells that harbor an innate intelligence. So talk to your cells. Tell them, with singularity of conviction, that they are healed.

Believe and you will heal.

THE ENGIMA OF HEALING

So how does Energy Medicine work? According to Robert Becker, M.D.,[10] twice-nominated for a Nobel Prize, when the limb of a salamander is amputated, it regenerates itself completely. When this same amputation is performed on a frog, the frog is unable to grow a new limb because the frog does not go through the process of **dedifferentiation**. Dedifferentiation is defined as the capacity to transform the energy circuitry from mature to primitive cells. In Dr. Becker's research, he discovered that in post-status amputation, the amputated limbs create a positive electrical charge for 2-3 days. The frog retains the positive charge. As a result, it can not undergo dedifferentiation; hence, it cannot grow a new limb. However, the salamander undergoes a shift in negative electrical charges after two or three days. It then returns to baseline. As a result, it can regenerate the lost limb; the salamander has healed itself.

Humans have access to the same universal energy as the salamander. The potential for healing via dedifferentiation also is constantly available for our own healings. In the dynamics of human healing, dedifferentiation also happens because we have similar internal, direct electrical current systems (DC), like our friend the salamander.[11] In the process of energy-based healing, we switch from the digital brain system to the more primordial, analog system. Whenever we wish to heal, we switch from an information based, digital orientation and return to the hub of healing within our own primordial analog resources.

We need to get out of our heads and into our hearts. We move from thinking to feeling. I believe it is here that we generate the dedifferentiation of electrical charges for self-induced healing. Understanding this enigma of Energy Medicine, dedifferentiation, means we can shift from our mind-based skepticism to a belief-based consciousness. Socrates said, "Know thyself." I say, "Heal thyself."

Our contemporary analytical sciences demonstrate a preoccupation with predictability and consistency creating a non-dynamic world. As a society we tend to assume that our contemporary medical and scientific knowledge is infallible. Yet, according to an article in the *British Medical Journal* in 1991, 85% of medical treatments at that time had never been assessed at all.[12]

DEEP DYNAMIC SCIENCE

The soul is being incorporated in medicine under what I call **deep dynamic science**. This burgeoning model brings soul back to science. I believe that a conscious connection to Spirit provides the essential pathway for the re-emergence of Energy Medicine.

Energy Medicine is not founded on analytical thinking; it integrates intuition and vision in its application. For example, in his national best-seller, *Chaos: Making a New Science*, James Gleick provides fascinating insights into the inherent order that underlies the seemingly erratic and chaotic nature of our universe. Gleick coins the term the **Butterfly Effect** to describe our inseparability. In other words, the initial starting point has a significant impact on the output of the end point. For example, I believe that a butterfly that spreads its wings in an Amazon rain forest affects the weather patterns throughout metropolitan areas of the world.

Energy Medicine is being reborn in the new millennium. A paradigm shift is occurring. You can experience, not analyze, God. Magic, not logic, is becoming accepted. By magic, I mean those creative, unpredictable, imaginative forces that are now being acknowledged by various scientists. Profound advancements in the realm of physics are leading us to re-explore the dynamics of metaphysics. The wonder that was lost in the industrial age is now resurging in our collective consciousness. The energies of the mischievous deva, the philosopher king, the goddess and Gaia are reappearing in our daily lives in alternative healing practices, juxtaposed to medical prescriptions.

Herbert Benson, M.D., the founder and president of the Mind/Body Institute at Harvard Medical School, in *Timeless Healing: The Power and Biology of Belief*, discovers that we have a need for nourishment from faith. Under the vanguard of alternative medicine, bravehearts like Dr. Herbert Benson, Dr. Deepak Chopra, Dr. Andrew Weil, Dr. Dean Ornish, Dr. Carl Simonton, Dr. Larry Dossey, and many others are bringing soul to medicine.

The most interesting discovery I have found in the history of modem medicine is the relative absence of healing practices in medical literature. The truth is that healing, to become whole, is the core of medicine. Wholeness is synonymous with wellness. Prior to the current shift, medical schools rarely educated practitioners about holistic healing. Today more and more physicians and medical schools are exploring the mindbody connection.

THE HEART HAS REASON

In the old paradigm, the mindbody was the focus of the approach. In Energy Medicine, the heart is the center of healing as we evolve into the new millennium. When we go to a doctor, apart from our physical diagnosis, our belief system, support group and Mind-Made Medicine (which is based on internal communication, how we feel in our heart) is responsible for our total picture of health. In mechanical medicine, the doctor does not take all this into consideration, truncating many possibilities for recovery. According to Howard Beckman and Richard Frankel, the average general practitioner is with a patient approximately seven minutes. During sessions, doctors primarily talk rather than listen. In 1975, this time was eleven minutes per patient, and now, most doctors interrupt within the first 18 seconds of the patient's attempt to explain their initial complaint.

A nation-wide survey conducted over a five-year period by researchers at George Washington University School of Medicine on 5,000 acutely-ill patients (primarily cardiovascular patients), found the important variable related to critical survival was not prestige, sophisticated technology, or professional expertise – but the quality of compassion in nursing care. Patients who were held and reassured by the nurses evidenced the best outcomes.

The heart is the center of Energy Medicine. Our hearts know reasons that our mind cannot know. Are we aware that the human heart produces 2.5 watts of electromagnetic energy with each beat, which is enough to power a small radio or a bulb?

According to my colleague, geologist Sandy Sumich, quartz crystals, formed under differential pressure, are piezoelectric; that is, they have an electrical charge. I personally believe that human beings are also **piezoelectric**. The difference between a human being and a quartz crystal is that an outside pressure is required in their formation whereas human beings have an intrinsic "pressure," which is our inherent will.

THE WILL TO HEAL

One of the most essential ingredients in healing is the will to heal. Consciousness works as the catalyst that galvanizes our intrinsic will. It is interesting to note that the power of the will alone is insufficient. It must be coupled with surrender. Will is our warrior aspect. Surrender is the way of the lover. When will and surrender interface, we find our direction along our own Healer's Journey.

Why do some people heal while others do not? Healing happens when we allow it to happen. The combination of intention and will is prerequisite for healing. Intention means manifesting our conscious desires or passions. Will is conviction in action. If will and intention fail to marry, we lessen our potential to heal.

The mechanical model of medicine is based on the Newtonian science of cause-and-effect while the dynamics of synchronicity form the basis of Energy Medicine. **Synchronicity** can be defined as meaningful coincidences where Spirit speaks to us. When we attract synchronicity in the moment, we go beyond the limitations of a cause and effect reality. The more we attract synchronicity, the more we will experience the magic and miracles of energy-based healing.

In the advent of Energy Medicine, the pineal gland will be used as a directive for the healer. According to my understanding, the pineal gland will grow in the new millennium. As we are going through the collective shift in consciousness, our pineal gland (our "third eye") will evolve. The pineal gland represents a doorway to the direct perception of intuitive understanding.

MAPPING ENERGY

In order to document energy-based healing, I experimented, as a subject, with Kirlian photography. The Kirlian method is high-voltage imaging of luminous corona electrical discharge without the aid of a camera. Former UCLA researcher, Thelma Moss, Ph.D., author of *The Body Electric*, referred me to John Hubacher who performed a series of tests before and after I administered energy healing. The results demonstrated that the electrical discharge from my hands significantly increased after energy based healing. This means of graphically representing the human emission of bioenergy may help us in discovering and detecting diseases.

RELEASING CELLULAR MEMORY

It is a basic tenet of Energy Medicine that human organs metabolize emotions and store them as cellular memories in the major organs of the body. The lungs fossilize sadness; the spleen stores melancholy; the kidneys hold fear; the heart harbors the shock of extreme emotions; and anger and resentment are metabolized in the liver. If you experience problems with a specific organ, it may be helpful, along with more traditional allopathic treatments, to actively address the cellular memory of the organ-specific emotions. In our process of healing, traumatic memories are replaced by their complementary emotional energies.

For example, in my own experience on the Healer's Journey, when my lungs and kidneys were breaking down, I had to come out of sadness (lungs) and fear (kidneys) vibrations by reaching out and offering healing to others. When I realized the whole world was my home, I was able to transform my pulmonary-stored sadness into joy, and my renal-based fear into courage by embracing the world. Transforming cellular memories is one of the keys to Energy Medicine:

Where there is a minus bring a plus.

The cover story of Time (May 12, 1997) featured Andrew Weil, M.D., who prescribed a health menu. In Dr. Weil's "Do's and Don'ts," he says, "…reach out to someone from whom you're estranged." Often our patterns of fear and our projections and judgments cause us to distance ourselves from friends and family. Healing fragmented relationships is often like bringing back lost pieces of our hologram.

Wholeness also can be initiated in reverse, that is the world comes to the individual. In the Hawaiian Kahuna tradition, when a person has a breakdown, the Kahuna healer gathers the entire community and asks for a ritual of forgiveness, where each member of the group is asked to let go of all and any resentment that they are holding against the ailing person. Then the healing takes place.

How To Apply Energy Medicine

Forgiveness is the first element of Energy Medicine. It is by forgiving that we let go of our past traumatic cellular memories. My healing was enhanced when Louise Hay gave me a blue card that said: "the past is over," and I started to carry it with me every day. Everything we are is because of everything that was. We heal when we let go of our past.

The second step in practicing Energy Medicine is to allow synchronicity to be our guiding light. When we have scarcity, disease and negativity, we first must be willing to become trusting. That is, realizing that the world is for us, not against us. We then begin to attract meaningful coincidences in our everyday life. When we become aware of synchronicity, we break the mechanical chain of cause-and-effect.

Breathing is the third key. Life originates with breath, and breath circulates life anew. In 1931, Otto Warburg, M.D., Nobel laureate found that cancer metabolism is correlated with a lack of oxygen to human cells. So whenever we are bombarded with information, overwhelmed by emotion, or exhausted, try pausing. Take a deep breath… and exhhhhhale.

No academic degree is necessary for practicing Energy Medicine. Anyone can practice Energy Medicine by listening to the language of their body and the voice of their soul. There is not just one way in the kingdom of healing. There are as many ways to use Energy Medicine as there are people who wish to practice it. We are the greatest healers. We can heal ourselves from anything. For our readership, we outline the following specific steps as a guide to incorporating Energy Medicine in daily living.

A Bird's Eye View of Energy Medicine

We will introduce *Mind-Made Medicine* in *Chapter Three* where we will learn to create our own walking talking internal pharmacies. Our internal and external dialogues generate potent psychophysiological changes. We need to acknowledge the tremendous power of our thoughts and emotions. We are responsible for every thought and emotion we choose to hold. The very words we utter on a daily basis create the reality of our health.

Here is an example of something we can do to begin accessing this healing. The next time we feel heavy-hearted or under-the-weather, take a break from whatever we are doing, go to a mirror, and change our expression into what we desire. (Mirror, mirror on the wall, who is the _____ of them all?, and we fill in the blank!). Tell ourself we are the best. We will be surprised that by changing our facial language into our desires, our bodies and immune systems will listen, and change accordingly.

Foods that Heal is the next step and is addressed in *Chapter Four.*

We must learn to honor our bodies by nourishing and healing our cells with nutraceuticals, that is, when food itself becomes medicine. This is a new way of looking at food. We need to view food as a healing ally versus treating it as a routine or as the enemy. Often I have learned in my healing practices that when we feel blocked, either emotionally and/or physically, our stomach is the first thing affected. Taking ginger tea can remedy nausea, as well as migraine headaches.

We not only take in food, we also take in sound that can be used as a powerful vibrational tool to create soothing effects that enhance healing. In Chapter Five, we will cover *Hear and Your Soul Shall Live*. Everyone is born with their own harmonics, the human voice producing two or more notes simultaneously. Our own voice, with its particular resonance, is readily available to use as an instrument of peace. Try this. Inhale deeply using your stomach muscles. Then create a prolonged "aaaaahhhh…" aloud while exhaling. The effect of this simple dose of sound medicine may surprise us (minimally, it may induce a laugh or two!).

The Biology of Environment will be discussed in *Chapter Six, Earth Medicine*. Our surroundings have a tremendous impact on our health and well-being. We often are unaware of the power of **geopathic stress** (GS), the negative effect of earth. If we live in an area with limited space, either spend more time outdoors or invite Mother Nature to come indoors and live with us.

If we cannot incorporate the above tools of transformation, we can always learn to laugh. The far-reaching impact of *Amuse-ology* will be explored in *Chapter Seven*. The role of humor is becoming recognized in such settings as hospitals and business offices. We recommend a healthy dose of humor in the home, giggles in the garage, and chuckles in church. The aforementioned meditation-at-the-mirror in and of itself may provide the very stimulus we need to try a sample of amuse-medicine.

Reality is not objective. We author our reality. The world around us is changed when we alter our perception of it. *Healing the Healer* in *Chapter Eight* will help us to intentionally show that we are healthy *when we see things as we would like them to be, not as they are.* For example, when someone seems difficult to get along with and we feel that it is jeopardizing our health, either emphasize the valuable things that person has done for us, or we need to free ourselves from the relationship.

We live in a world of possibilities. These opportunities become readily accessible the first moment we recognize Spirit in something, someone or somewhere. *Chapter Nine: The Spirit of Possibilities*, will open us to the **hologram** – the part is contained in the whole, and the whole is contained in the part. In our interactions, we can focus on the bigger picture rather than on the immediate situation. For example, if we are trying to find a place to rent, we need to visualize our perfect home, in depth, and then hold the holographic image to help manifest our vision.

Albert Einstein once said, "There are only two ways to live your life. One is as though nothing is a miracle. The other is as though everything is a miracle." The miracle of energy happens when we allow it to flow. There is a perpetual dilemma between the mind and the soul. To bridge this chasm between reason and emotion, between logic and magic, we need to flow. Everything in the world is "meaning-*full*" when we open ourselves to energy. Otherwise it is all hieroglyphics.

The flow of energy is the River of Life.

EXERCISES FOR TRANSFORMATION AND HEALING

1. **Forgiveness**: Each night find a quiet moment before we fall asleep. Say, "I thank you for this day. I forgive the one who has upset me the most today. Kindly help me to see something precious this person has done. I am willing to release all of these things." Practicing this can bring a sense of gratitude that promotes healing.

2. **Attracting Synchronicity**: As we start opening our hearts to synchronicity, other hearts will synchronize with us and we will begin to experience harmony. Actively picture someone in our hearts. If we receive a letter or phone call from them around the same time, tell them about this "coincidence." This focus will open the door and allow synchronicity to continue to flow in.

3. **Breathing**: Place one hand on our stomach, and rhythmically and slowly feel our hand moving out as we exhale, and feel our hand moving in as we inhale. Become aware of our abdominal breathing, our "second heart," rather than mechanically breathing from our chest. We can use this technique anywhere, in the car, in the bath, while waiting in line in a store, etc. This will enhance our awareness of our connection to the cosmic breath.

4. **Soul Food**: A healthy body is a healthy mind. It is very helpful to respect the body by fasting periodically and going out into the sun, drinking fresh-squeezed vegetable juices, and giving and receiving a lot of love. Regular exercise, such as walking, can be fun with someone we enjoy.

5. **Sound Health**: Find a moment everyday away from all distractions. Lie down on our back. Surrender. Become aware of breathing, and listen to the sound of silence. Practice nonjudgment as we allow our body and mind to receive the sound health of silence.

6. **Earth Healing**: Bring something sacred into our home, or into the home of someone we love, as an offering, such as a flower, a fallen leaf, a feather, or a flame of a candle.

7. **Celebrate Energy**: Do at least one thing each day that demonstrates our appreciation for the life energy around us. Record this daily in a personal notebook of thanks. For example, find something that represents power and sacredness.

Notes

1. Genesis 2:7, New Testament: "And the Lord formed man from the dust of the ground and breathed into his nostrils the breath of life, and man became a living being."

2. The Sanskrit word meaning *life force.*

3. The dantian, according to the ancient healing art, Qi'gong, is located about two inches below the navel.

4. The subtle energies flow through our veins, **nadis**, which became the meridian in Chinese traditional medicine. Mobilizing this energy along our marma points (Indian tradition) and acupuncture points (Chinese practice) is the main practice of healing.

5. An excellent reference is *The Way of the Qigong: The Art and Science of Chinese Energy* Healing by Kenneth Cohen.

6. Bhagavad Gita 2:23.

7. Refer to *Prayer is Good Medicine: How to Reap the Healing Benefits of Prayer* by Larry Dossey, M.D..

8. Researched in *The Conscious Universe: The Scientific Truth of Psychic Phenomena* by Dean Radin, Ph.D..

9. This will be further explored in Chapter 3: Mind-Made Medicine: Walking Talking Pharmacy.

10. Author of *Cross Currents: The Perils of Electropollution, The Promise of Electromedicine.*

11. The salamander is my symbol and reminder of Heal Thyself. Use and give away salamander pins freely. Salamanders are our angels of the new millenium.

12. *British Medical Journal* #303, pp. 798-799.

❦

CHAPTER III

MIND-MADE MEDICINE

Walking Talking Pharmacy

'Tis the mind that makes the body rich.

— Shakespeare

In the *Rebirth of Energy Medicine*, we introduced specific steps to applying Energy Medicine in our daily lives. This chapter details practical ways of creating our own internal pharmacies that we can access in our efforts to heal ourselves. **Psychoneuroimmunology (PNI)** addresses the communication link between our behavior, our nervous system and our immune processes. In Energy Medicine, there is **mindbody**; there is no separation. Steven Locke, M.D., a professor at Harvard Medical School, calls the mindbody approach the third revolution in Western medicine, the first being surgery, and the second, penicillin. The chemical language of emotion and the immune system is neuropeptides. These **neuropeptides** are remarkably illuminated by Professor Candace Pert, Ph.D., of Georgetown University Medical Center in her authoritative book *Molecules of Emotion: The Science Behind Mind-Body Medicine*. These molecules communicate with our entire body. They are protein sequences that are the building blocks of DNA.[1]

THE UNIVERSAL LANGUAGE OF PEPTIDES

Peptides are not only protein sequences, they are charged with intelligence, the same inherent, omnipresent intelligence contained in nature. In 1982 at Washington University, biologists Drs. Orians and Rhoades conducted an interesting experiment with neighboring tree species, alder and willow. One set of trees was experimentally infected with webworms and caterpillars. The infected group rallied to protect themselves. They altered their protein counts, and started secreting tannins and terpenes.

These secretions made the leaves inedible, the insects died, and the disease process ceased. In essence, the trees had healed themselves.

Perhaps even more fascinating is another finding. The uninfected neighboring trees (the control group in this study) seemed to receive a "message" from infected trees. As a result they also began producing tannins and terpenes, protecting themselves from infection. From dolphins to trees, such communication represents the ubiquitous and intelligent language of peptides, awaiting our understanding.

THE MODERN BIRTH OF MIND-MADE MEDICINE

George F. Solomon, M.D., the contemporary father of Mind-Made Medicine, coined the term **psychoimmunology** to describe the link between our mind and our immune system. Robert Ader, Ph.D., later expanded the term to PNI to highlight the importance of the nervous system and its relationship to the immune system.

Dr. Solomon's research emphasized the relationship between personality, behaviors and immunology. He outlined immune-competent personality traits: finding meaning in our work, expressing anger constructively, asking for favors and support from family and friends and the ability to deal with difficult people with ease.[2] Dr. Solomon later discovered links between personality style and disease (e.g., rheumatoid arthritis, cancer, AIDS). For example, a "nice guy" personality constellation was significantly correlated with rheumatoid arthritis (a disorder characterized by immuno-compromise) and unassertive behavior patterns. Dr. Solomon even found that mice who demonstrated fighting behaviors had stronger immune systems, hence, his quote "…it is good for your health to express anger…, even if you are a mouse."[3]

LOVE AND IMMUNOLOGY

A whole orchestra of healing hormones and a dance of electrical impulses occur within our immune system when we are in love. We can reach euphoria and peak energy by creating a powerful substance, **phenylethylamine** (PEA). PEA is an important psycho-regulator that works as a natural stimulant, like amphetamine, in our bodies. It is essential for our well-being. The joy of beauty is love, and the beauty of PEA is joy. We can even manufacture PEA in the anticipation of love when the object of love is absent. It is interesting to note that chocolate, cheddar cheese and salami also promote the production of PEA.[4] Yet when we have the real thing, love — salami, cheese and chocolate can go back on our diet docket.

David McClelland, Ph.D., a Harvard psychologist, explored the psychobiology of love. When we have a cold, apart from other therapies, try the therapy of love. Dr. McClelland stated that, "Now, when I'm getting a cold I spend some time thinking about loving relationships. A couple of times it even stopped my cold."[5] In other words, we can imagine, in our minds and hearts, a time when we were in love. This visualization may help reduce our cold symptoms. Just the imagery of love activates our immune system, and perhaps an angel of PEA will alight.

There is no scarcity of love. We do not have to have an external object of love, we can find that love within. There are countless ways to enhance our self-esteem. Gloria Steinem calls self-esteem "a revolution from within." For example, we can wear a favorite pin, a scarf, or a dress and look in the mirror and say "I love you." We also can have love and romance with life in general by following our dreams.

Our perceptions of love affect our health. In a 35-year longitudinal study coordinated by Drs. Stanley King, Harry Russek, Gary Schwartz, et al., it was found that 91% of the participant students from Harvard who felt they lacked an affectionate relationship with their mothers in childhood developed serious health problems in the middle interim of their lives.

Janice Kiecolt-Glaser, Ph.D.,[6] and Ronald Glaser, Ph.D., discovered that "feeling" lonely significantly related to immune system compromises. When students were preparing for examination, those students who "felt" lonely had the least active **natural killer** cells (NK). NK cells also preprogrammed to help fight viral infections and metastatic cancer. In Mind-Made Medicine, it is our perception of our experiences that either helps or hinders our immune system.

THE HEALING OF COMMUNITY

Roseto is an Italian-American town in eastern Pennsylvania. Since 1882, residents there have enjoyed a strong sense of community. Their diets and lifestyles were not according to Hoyle (i.e., they included high fat and high calorie consumption). However, the incidence of cardiovascular and other diseases was low due to communal eating and other family rituals. When we share our life, our joys and sorrows, in the warmth of community it seems to protect us from negative health factors. We can call this the *Roseto Effect*. In recent generations, with the fragmentation of the family unit, disease rates in Roseto are now comparable with neighboring communities.

A sense of community works as a buffer. In the Japanese way of life, a similar sense of community and festive group activities are partly responsible for their longevity. The Japanese idea of **amae** describes the protective nature of goodwill with the group. Dr. Leonard Syme,[7] epidemiologist from the University of California, Berkeley, links amae's effect to the fine health enjoyed by family-oriented Japanese who maintain strong family ties even after migrating to the United States. Not only does diet promotes Japanese longevity but amae also plays a part.

HEART AND HEALING

Dean Ornish, M.D., author of *Love and Survival: The Scientific Basis for the Healing Power of Intimacy* (1998) has demonstrated the health benefits of opening our hearts in reversing heart disease. Dr. Ornish prescribed a low-fat diet, change in lifestyle, exercise and, most importantly, relating to others lovingly, as ways to promote survival. After one year, Dr. Ornish demonstrated that chest pains significantly dissipated, and arterial clogging had reversed in over 82% of patients without using drugs and surgery. *Newsweek* called these results "revolutionary." Dr. Ornish emphasized the role of intimacy and love as the most meaningful intervention, typically neglected in the medical profession.[8]

Thomas Oxman, M.D., and a team of researchers at Dartmouth Medical School highlight another interesting aspect of heart and healing. They found that after open heart surgery, patients who felt comforted by their religious beliefs had a survival rate three times greater than those who did not. Of these patients, those who also reported being involved in community activities and faith had a survival rate ten times greater.[9]

THE HEALING POWER OF "P"

The easiest way to bring the healing power of connectedness into everyday living is by having at least one "P" in our lives: person, plant or pet. When we feel lonely and isolated, our immune system becomes suppressed.

In order for the healing juices of the immune system to flow, we need to have supportive people in our lives. For example, having a friend who we can call in the middle of the night, and say, "I can't believe this shit happened to me!" Just having someone there who we can rely on, and who will listen to us without judgment, provides a valuable boost to our immune systems. We are brought up in a society where fear of abandonment abounds. This basic fear prevents us from connecting with others, and triggers immune-suppressive responses throughout our body. Jean-Paul Sartre was incorrect when he said: *the* other *is hell.* Others can be a tremendous boost to our well-being.

If we feel a twinge of misanthropy come over us, we might instead consider adopting a plant. I never leave my house without talking to my friends, the gardenia and night-blooming jasmine. When I return, I always share how my day was with them. Ellen Langer, Ph.D., Professor of Psychology at Harvard University, conducted a fabulous study. In 1976 in a nursing home, a group of elderly residents were given house plants to care for. In a comparison group, nursing staff attended to the plants. After 1½ years, the survival rate of the patients caretaking for their plants was twice that of the control group patients.

Taking care of a plant gives us a sense of responsibility, and talking to a plant gives us a sense of connection. Research scientist Cleve Backster demonstrated that plants do have consciousness, which he calls **primary perception**. That is, plants not only share a basic nonlocal intelligence but they also share an ability to communicate in nonverbal terms.

If we do not have time for plant-talk, welcome a three-letter angel of love: p-e-t. Pet connections work as a living sedative and can lower our blood pressure. We benefit from sharing our heart with an animal — whether it be a swan or a salamander, a Siamese or a sheltie.

Psychiatrist Erika Friedmann, M.D., from the University of Pennsylvania, discovered that this pet-love gave people a stronger reason to live than family and spouses. The underlying reason is that animals show us unconditional love. They always greet us affectionately no matter how long we have been gone or what our mood du jour may be. Our tendency to be judgmental and conditional with ourselves and others interrupts the flow of love. Even conversations with a goldfish or a golden retriever can promote coronary health.

WRITING OUR WAY TO HEALTH

When we cannot make a connection outside our selves, as outlined above, we can make a connection within. There is always hope. We are never completely alone. Writing our way to health is a technique for stimulating our minds, hearts and immune systems. Psychologist James Pennebaker, Ph.D., from Southern Methodist University found that writing about our traumas for 20 minutes weekly for four weeks can significantly improve our immune systems (a control group wrote about general life events in the same time period). Dr. Pennebaker compared blood samples before and after the writing experiment. The group who recorded their traumas had fewer symptoms and made fewer trips to the doctor.

In 1989, David Spiegel, M.D., at Stanford School of Medicine, published his surprising results in the prominent British medical journal *The Lancet*.[10] Dr. Spiegel divided a group of female patients with metastatic breast cancer in two groups. Both groups were given identical medical treatments. The only differential variable was that patients within one group were assigned to a 90-minute weekly support group where they cried, cheered, and shared their stories within the safety of the group. In a five-year follow-up, the support group attendees had twice the lifespan of nonattending patients.

Isolation is contraindicated. Connection heals. We are all in this together. The language of the heart can be understood even without a single word being uttered.

SOMATIZATION THROUGH THE AGES

Soma comes from the Greek word that means body. People living in a particular era create a collective impression of what defines wellness and illness, which in turn manifests in patterns of disease. We somatize; our thoughts become realized in our bodies.

Every age has its own collective thought pattern based on the material advancements and values of the society. These cultural thought patterns have a far reaching impact on health trends.

For example, in the nineteenth century, prominent figures in literature and the arts romanitcized suffering and dying young. The incidence and prevalence of consumption (tuberculosis) increased as people accepted and adopted this paradigm.

Eventually, the collective consciousness changed, and the disease changed. Death at a young age was no longer glorified. The advent of the industrial revolution not only brought advancements in medicine; it also encouraged individuals to abandon their relative isolation and join with the progress of society.

Modern allopathic medicine is predicated on a disease-based model. Billions of dollars annually are invested to treat illness on a secondary and tertiary basis. In contrast, in ancient Chinese medicine, doctors were paid as long as the person remained healthy. Payments stopped and the doctors were fired when disease appeared. Our approach to energy-based medicine rejuvenates the ancient wisdom where medicine is health oriented versus disease-focused.

SPONTANEOUS REMISSION

From prehistoric time to the present, nature has provided us with mechanisms to self-repair, to self-heal spontaneously. Even the simplest cell has the capacity to repair its own genes. Trees demonstrate this inherent ability. Animals and amphibians share the same gift of spontaneous remission.

We can utilize this built-in intelligence from nature whenever we need to heal. Rockefeller University researcher, Rene Dubos, Ph.D., purports, "…probably 90% to 95% of the ailments for which people seek medical attention would take care of themselves without any medical help."[11] I believe every disease, including different types of cancer, can be healed by tapping into this spontaneous remission mechanism. Saint Augustine said, "Miracles do not happen in contradiction of nature, but in contradiction of what we know about nature."

In 1993, researchers Brenden O'Regan and Caryle Hirshberg published the largest collection of spontaneous remission cases (3,500). This remarkable collection, entitled *Spontaneous Remission: An Annotated Bibliography*, synthesizes research from over 830 medical journals in more than 20 languages.

The phenomenon of spontaneous healing has not been incorporated into main-stream medicine, to date. Healing happens all the time, and healing happens all over the world. Wherever faith goes, spontaneous healing can follow. Andrew Weil, M.D., suggests that, as more people believe in spontaneous healing, people will experience it more frequently.

People with "terminal" cancer, "incurable" diseases and people on crutches heal themselves. Every year more than five million people go to experience this healing miracle at a Roman Catholic shrine in Lourdes, France. The medical review board of Lourdes has scientifically documented hundreds of these healings.

Based on a synthesis of international research findings, the ingredients of spontaneous healing generally remain amorphous. In the *Heart of Healing*, published by the Institute of Noetic Sciences with William Poole, the following are some of the causative factors that are elegantly encapsulated:

1. **Favorable psychosocial change:** Charles Weinstock, a professor at Albert Einstein College of Medicine in New York, explored the mechanisms of spontaneous remission. He found that a positive psychosocial change (e . g., religious conversion, reconciliation in relationships , etc.) often occurred one to three weeks prior to the remission.

2. **Dramatic shift in life viewpoint:** Dr. Yujiro lkerni also discovered, at Kyushu University in Japan, that individuals who experienced spontaneous remission frequently had undergone a dramatic, positive change in their outlook on life.

3. **Less depression, less trusting of medical diagnoses, autonomy, and stronger support systems.** Dr. Marco de Vries of the Netherlands discovered that healed patients were less depressed and had greater autonomy. They tended to feel less trusting about following medical advice, and enjoyed greater social support.

I believe, as a result, these patients experienced a radical existential shift. When we go through an instant transformation from feeling powerless to feeling empowered, we facilitate our healing process.

At the turn of the 19th century, Sir William Osler said, "It is much more important to know what sort of patient has the disease than what sort of disease the patient has." In my healing practice, I have repeatedly witnessed that it is not the disease but our attitude, belief, coping skills, support system, and lifestyle that enable the miracle of healing. Spontaneous healing is nature's gift to us. Mark Twain once joked about it, "Nature heals and the doctor sends the bill." Each and every human being is born with uniqueness, which is our life purpose.[12]

This is our song. Find it, and heal.

Whenever we want to heal, we need to return to the home of our own hearts to kindle the flame of passion within, something or someone we naturally love. Here we reunite with our purpose in life, which contains the entire score for our healing and happiness. The song can be any thing, a sport, a dream, a hobby, an animal, anything that makes our heart sing. Dis-ease breaks us. The song of life heals us. God lives in our hearts. When we follow our song, we summon the energy to take a leap into the open arms of God... to surmount any obstacle and become whole.

The Sky Is Partly Bright

It is our *interpretation* of our health status that produces our desired results. For example, in Alameda County, California, approximately 7,000 people completed a questionnaire rating their view of their health. Their actual health was not the significant factor. Rather it was their *perception* of their health that mattered. In a nine-year follow-up, men who rated their health as poor had a death rate 2.3 times as great as men who rated their health as excellent. Among female subjects, the morbidity rate was five times greater![13] The next time someone asks us about our health, let us apply this technique, and emphasize our well-being. This mobilizes the healing medicines in our minds. "So how is your health?" "Great! Wonderful!" We are practicing positive perceptions that promote PNI.

Crucial factors in generating Mind-Made Medicine are our tendency to perceive ourselves as being hope-full rather than hope-less, and power-full as opposed to power-less. Our words directly reflect our attitudes and perceptions. Words have tremendous power. They work like magnets, attracting to us what we create in our minds. The impact of this dynamic occurs with words spoken aloud, as well as with the vocabulary of our private, internal dialogues.

In a wonderful book entitled *Healthy Pleasures* by Robert Ornstein, Ph.D., and David Sobel, M.D., the authors cite several interesting studies that are highlighted here. In one example, a group of female patients were awaiting the results of their cervical biopsies. There was a significant correlation between the women's use of negative words and poor test results. That is, women whose choice of words emphasized negative emotions and/ or ideas (e.g., "dark, difficult," or "disgusting" depicting a discouragement with life) were more likely to receive unfavorable test results indicative of cervical cancer. In contrast, women who used positive words (e.g., "longing, wish," and "desire," reflecting a zest for living) were more likely to receive favorable results.

In my seminars, I ask participants to quickly respond to the question, "How is the weather today?" When a person answers "partly cloudy," it indicates that the power of their words have not been fully realized. We then work together until they experience a shift in perception where they report that the sky is "partly sunny." It is interesting to note that in our popular media, this "partly sunny sky" orientation is rarely portrayed.[14]

Some of us may experience difficulties instantly changing our self-talk. We need to recognize the importance and power of this internal dialogue and commit to change. We stimulate PNI when we observe and practice acts of kindness. David McClelland, Ph.D., calls this the *Mother Teresa Effect*.[15] In an interesting study, students viewed a film of Mother Teresa working in India. The results from follow-up blood samples revealed that a significant marker, salivary immunoglobulin antigen (SIgA), was elevated. SIgA protects us from upper respiratory tract infections, and symptoms such as coughs and colds. So the next time we feel under-the-weather, we can watch a heart-warming movie, or better yet, go out and extend our hearts in an act of kindness to another.

How To Practice Mind-Made Medicine

We have seen clearly in this chapter that our minds literally create a powerful pharmacy, the hormones, neuropeptides, and innumerable unnamed biochemicals, that move and rejuvenate us as is intended by the intelligence of nature.

Faith heals. Belief activates the neural pathways of healing. Healing is the gift of life. Our DNA contains the blueprint for healing. When we receive life-enhancing messages, such as "I love myself," we activate our circuitry of healing. Our mind and our cells are constantly communicating. Let us be aware of these life lines of communication. This Mind-Made Medicine sends chemical messages to stimulate our genes to repair our ailing DNA.

The communication in the mind happens by path ways that are nerve endings separated by synaptic gaps. The nerve endings have dendrites that are not anatomically connected. It is by the intensity of electrical impulses that we bridge the gap of dendrites and activate the healing mechanism of Mind-Made Medicine.

It is our intentions, choices and actions that propel us toward health. In this chapter, we have reviewed specific, practical ways to heal: opening our souls, attracting love, connecting with P's, finding our song of life, creating hopefull-ness and power-full-ness, and involvement with acts of kindness and faith.

> *Dis-ease is a sense of loss.*
> *Healing is sense of power.*

What can we do to begin our healing at this very moment? We can start in our relationships and our jobs. Whenever we feel dis-ease, we can choose to change. We can bring power by connecting to any "P." When we connect with plants, pets or people we trigger the healing pathways. Connection is the mechanism where we return to life instinct, **eros**, creating the pharmacy to heal and experiencing its rejuvenating power.

If we have critical people around us, we need to bring supportive, nonjudgmental people into our lives. Compassion versus criticism accelerates our healing. Criticism does not promote change. Compassion encourages change. We can benefit from spending time with cheerful people because their energies will help elevate our perceptions.

By bringing positive vibrations into our lives, we heal.

Ancient wisdom teaches us:

As a man thinketh in his heart, so is he.[16]

EXERCISES FOR TRANSFORMATION AND HEALING

1. **Empowering Peptides**: A single touch, an uplifting story, a pat on the back, and a loving look all travel in the form of peptides that activate our inherent healing system. Let us nurture ourselves by giving ourselves a pat on the back each morning when we arise, and each night before we sleep. It is okay. If we cannot swim with a dolphin, we can attract dolphin-like people, people who are cheerful and playful, into our lives. Bring the flow of peptides.

2. **PNI Talk**: We can change the critical way we talk to ourselves into self-talk that promotes our self-esteem. For example, when we doubt ourselves, remember that we are powerful creators. We can reinforce this belief by repeating, "I am capable and creative."

3. **Love is the Drug**: We can bring lots of love into our everyday living. Let us begin by nurturing our own hearts. We can mail ourselves a valentine any time of the year saying "I Love You." In fact, it will be very health-full to do this often throughout the year as a reminder of the benefit of the "I Love You" drug.

4. **Song of Life**: Whether or not we can sing on tune, each of us has a song that we are born with. This song is actually any form of inner "gift" or talent. We are good for something. Find and practice these hidden talents.

5. **Partly Bright Sky**: When life seems miserable, we can find one ray of hope in the midst of the storm. For example, if our car does not start, instead of cursing, let us praise it for how wonderfully it has served us on uncountable occasions. On days we feel down on ourselves, we can select one positive thing to focus on throughout that day (e.g., "I have nice eyes," or "My pet is always good to me"). It can be most helpful to choose

something that spontaneously makes us laugh (e.g., "I have the most unusual nose in the world," or "I give so much to others, I should be Santa Claus!").

6. **A Dose of Kindness**: Let us begin with ourselves. Take five extra minutes today and listen to a favorite song, or eat a favorite food. Allow 15-30 minutes extra to commune with the sandman. During this time we can clear our minds of clutter. When we go out, we can also practice kindness with others. This can be especially fun when we do it anonymously. For example, find a parking meter that has expired, and feed it a coin or two (please do this at your own risk and responsibility). Recall that we can also derive health benefits from looking at a movie or book that depicts the milk of human kindness.

Notes

1. The dynamics of DNA will be further elaborated later in this chapter.

2. *Natural Health*, January-February 1992.

3. *Immune and Nervous System Interactions: An Analytic Bibliography Supporting Key Postulates on Communication Links, Similarities, and Implications*, 1996.

4. In 1991, a British study reported that the average person consumed 16 pounds of chocolate in that year. Was there a link to PEA?

5. In *The Healer Within*, Steven Locke, M.D., and Douglas Colligan, p. 242.

6. Janice K. Kiecolt-Glaser is a clinical health psychologist specializing in psychoneuroimmunology and Director of the Ohio State University Institute for Behavioral Medicine Research. Her research on stress associated with caregiving and marital relationships has been featured in many news outlets.

7. S. Leonard Syme is a Professor of Epidemiology and Community Health (Emeritus) in the School of Public Health at UC Berkeley whose research focuses on the relationship between health and such psychosocial factors as poverty, stress and social isolation.

8. Refer to *Dr. Dean Ornish's Program for Reversing Heart Disease: The Only System Scientifically Proven to Reverse Heart Disease without Drugs or Surgery* by Dean Ornish, M.D.

9. *Psychosomatic Medicine*, 1995. To learn more about Thomas Oxman, M.D., see *https://worldwidehumanitarian.com/2019/07/11/thomas-oxman/*

10. See Spiegel, David, M.D., "Effect of Psychosocial Treatment on Survival of Patients with Metastatic Breast Cancer," *The Lancet*, Volume 334, Issue 8668, 14 october 1989, pp. 888-89.

11. Refer to *The Healing Brain: A Scientific Reader*, edited by Robert Ornstein and Charles Swencionis, p. 136

12. Psychotherapist Lawrence LeShan popularized "the life song" which he used successfully in his clinical practice with cancer patients.

13. *American Journal of Epidemiology*, 1983.

14. I would like to have a television show that has the theme, "the sky is partly bright." Instead of talking about accidents and disasters, it will talk about the child who is born eight pounds healthy, and in my back yard even the cactus had a flower, and two neighbors who never spoke with one another spoke today.

15. Original study is "The effect of motivational arousal through films on salivary immunoglobulin A," by David C. McClelland & Carol Kirshnit, *Psychology & Health*, Volume 2, Issue 1 1988.

16. Proverbs 23:7

PART TWO

HEALING THE BODY

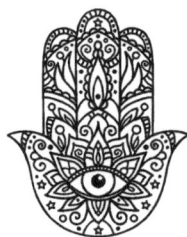

❀

CHAPTER IV

FOOD THAT HEALS

Rejuvenating the Body

Let food be thy medicine.

— Hippocrates

The evolution of humankind and the history of food are inseparable. Since the moment the sunflower first turned its face
toward the sun, humankind has been fascinated with witnessing the
unfolding of nature's love play. Shamanism was intimately linked with
the trees and plants, the givers of Life. The local flora and fauna were
respected as being endowed with guardian spirits. This knowledge is
re-emerging as **ethnobotany**, the healing relationship between plants
and people.[1]

In India, the goddess of food, **Annapurna**, was elevated to the
status of a symbolic deity. To this day, many Indian people perform
a ritualistic offering to Annapurna before eating. As industrializa-
tion has increased, mealtime prayer has gradually lost its meaning,
yet a deep reverence for food endures. Coconut milk, pristine, pure
and untouched, was thought of as a sacred offering to the gods. It
was used in celebrations of initiation, like the western tradition of
opening champagne.

THE MYTH, MAGIC AND MYSTERY OF PLANTS

Some plants became tools for white magic. For example, garlic
was used to exorcise evil spirits. Hot, piquant dry red peppers (the
basis of cayenne[2]) similarly were believed to ward off black magic.

Strings of red peppers still hang on the lintels of many Catholic shrines in the southwestern United States.[3] Although we now associate it exclusively with Christmas, mistletoe used to be hung year-round as an aegis to ward off misfortune. In India, limes have been used for this same purpose.

At the time of the pharaohs in Egypt, the onion was the symbol of the universe. Its layers represented the unfolding of mysteries on many levels. The papyrus plant, internally fashioned as a triangle, became honored for sharing the geometry of the pyramids. In my sojourn in Egypt, I learned that a papyrus amulet is still used today as a symbol of long life.

In ancient Greek mythology, plants and trees were considered bridges to the gods. It was believed that the oak leaves were conduits for divine will. Priests traveled to a northwestern region of Greece to ascertain celestial prophesies and teachings amongst the forests' rustling oak leaves.

In the Judea-Christian *Bible*, Moses' conversion occurred in his experience of the burning bush; the plant was afire yet not consumed. This bush became an oracle of God.

Jesus' miracle of loaves and fishes became a symbol of abundance through faith. When Christ shared food at the last supper, the breaking of bread became one of the seven holy sacraments.

NUTRACEUTICALS AS MODERN MEDICINE

> *The Lord has created medicines out of the earth;*
> *and he that is wise will not abhor them.*[4]

Mother Earth provides us with the healing power of food. In addition, modern technology has equipped us with a new line of nutrients based on amino acids, minerals, vitamins and herbs. The marriage of these resources gives birth to a hybrid called **nutraceuticals**.[5]

In our quest for health and healing, we may feel as though we are opening Pandora's box. We are flooded with multi-faceted, sometimes contradictory methodologies. Which approach or product do we choose to incorporate and which ones do we eschew? First, we can consult the healer within to determine which approach resonates best with our individual energy type. We can also consult our physician to clarify questions before instituting any of the following suggestions.

In this chapter, we will discuss food for the body, super-healing foods, and food for the soul.

Food is nature's intelligence manifest from the earth.

Based on our genetic characteristics, we can determine our focus. If we have a tendency for physical needs, incorporating **food for the body** will be most helpful. If our personal pace is frenzied, **super-healing foods** provide energizing and healing support. If we are highly-sensitive to subtle vibrations, then **food for the soul** is for us.

FOOD FOR THE BODY

Our bodies are sacred temples. Although this wisdom has ancient roots, and sounds familiar to many of us, reverent treatment of our temples in everyday practice remains alien. Our contemporary diets typically are characterized by image-fixated, high-stress, high-fat, high-sodium, high-sugar contents. Are we trashing our temples or are we worshipping them?

In my healing practice, I have repeatedly observed that unless a person is able to detoxify first, the optimal nutritional value of food is diminished. The first step toward creating a healthy body is cleansing our systems. Detoxification can be accomplished over a weekend or extended for one week. This can be continued periodically during the year, according to our needs and preferences.

It is helpful to drink fresh juices frequently (preferably vegetable juices) throughout our cleansing process. We should eliminate, or at least dramatically reduce, our intake of all cooked foods. After two or three days, we can begin to consume raw foods, and then we can gradually reintroduce cooked foods in the end-stage of detoxification. Cooked foods should be primarily whole grain foods: whole wheat, oats, brown rice, millet, couscous, quinoa, spelt, amaranth, and all types of dried beans.

Some natural forms of colonics can be utilized to enhance our process of purification. Medical genius, Max B. Gerson, M.D., inventor of the Gerson Therapy, suggested coffee enemas for purification. Anne Wigmore purports that a wheatgrass enema is highly-effective.[6]

Drinking wheatgrass juice during detoxification, as well as on a regular basis, is health-enhancing. Wheatgrass is chlorophyll-rich. What hemoglobin is to human blood, chlorophyll is to plant circulation. Just as hemoglobin carries oxygen to human cells, chlorophyll molecules transport oxygen to plant cells.[7] Drinking one ounce of wheatgrass juice is nutritionally equivalent to ingesting 2½ pounds of choice vegetables. It also contains abscisic acid that is found to shrink the size of tumors in animal studies.

If we feel resistant to using colonics, we alternatively can dissolve several spoonfuls of psyllium husks in juices, which provide enough fiber to enhance cleansing. We can drink this three times a day until detoxification is completed. Turkey rhubarb and slippery elm and other cleansing herbs that typically come in capsule form can be added to our regimen. Papaya, prunes, dates and figs are delicious, sweet cleansers. While completing our self detoxification, having a lymphatic-drainage massage will be beneficial. This type of massage promotes a clear lymph-flow toward the nodes. Earlier morning sunlight also facilitates our cleansing process.

The Virtue of Live Foods

According to Dr. Gerson, excessive sodium can cause hardening of the cell membranes, limiting the intra- and extra-cellular transport of nutrients. One change we can initiate is replacing sodium with a potassium rich diet. Removing salty, fatty, pickled and smoked foods from our diet can help remedy migraine headaches, tuberculosis, cancer, and other chronic diseases, according to Dr. Gerson.[7]

A healthy organism needs a high level of enzymes and minerals. In some foods, the application of heat destroys enzymes. Enzyme-depleted foods create a load on our system. Fatigue after a meal, constipation, feeling bloated, and headaches are all symptoms of enzyme depletion in our bodies.

Raw foods are the best source of minerals and enzymes. However, we cannot eat a dozen carrots every day (unless we aspire to be Bugs Bunny). However, we can juice them. Dr. Gerson was able to heal advanced cancer primarily by fresh carrot juice and other protocols. In his treatment, he found that only hydraulic press juicers[9] enable maximum preservation of live minerals and enzymes in the juicing process to facilitate the healing of cancer and many other diseases. Hydraulically-pressed juices go directly into the blood stream to feed our cells within a few minutes. In contrast, the average juicer works by a centrifugal mechanism that causes oxidization. As a result, enzymes and minerals are broken down, and their health benefits are reduced. If we cannot personally invest in a **Norwalk**, the Rolls Royce of juicers, we can still have access to enzyme-rich juices. Our local health food stores sell refrigerated juices that have been produced by the hydraulic method.

Our bodies are devised with selective uptake intelligence. That is, we are able to distinguish between beneficial and less beneficial food nutrients. When we primarily consume raw foods (e.g., juices, salads, fresh fruit and sprouts) we raise, on a cellular level, our microelectric potentials. Sprouts are a powerhouse of live energy. They are, on averge, four times as effective in their rate of absorption and enzymatic activity as compared to other raw foods. Our bodies naturally uptake beneficial molecules and eliminate toxic particles when this microelectric potential is elevated.

Our bioelectric intelligence is a vital part of Energy Medicine. Harry Oldfield and Roger Coghill, in their book *The Dark Side of the Brain: Major Discoveries in the Use of Kirlian Photography and Eloctrochrystal Therapy*, document various color reproductions of high-voltage Kirlian photography. Images of a whole food diet versus a typical fast-food diet reveal significant differences. Virtually no luminosity can be seen in images of the hands of subjects eating junk food in contrast to bright, radiating energies clearly seen from the hands of subjects eating healthy diets. Literally, we are what we eat.

pH IN ACTION

We are young as long as our cells are young. The quality of our blood determines the future of our health and disease. Robert Young, Ph.D., a microbiologist, has explored the relationship between mycotic infection (e.g., yeast, mold and fungus) and human disease. Our blood waste products from dietary intake include uric acid, lactic acid, acetate, alcohol and ethanol. In my personal experience, I was amazed that Dr. Young could differentiate between normal and abnormal cells in observing my live blood culture using a microscope. Here I also learned about the importance of maintaining an acid-alkaline balance.

In his book, *One Sickness, Disease, Treatment: Life and Death Are In the Blood*, Dr. Young suggests that a 4:1 alkaline to acid ratio (equivalent to pH=7.3) is optimal for healthy blood. Acids are neutralized in our systems by alkalis. For our readers, the following are examples of alkaline-producing foods: soy products, lima beans, vegetable juices, sprouts, flaxseeds, walnuts, millet and buckwheat. Acid-enhancing foods include all meats (including poultry and fish) and dairy products.

COMMON FOOD AND CANCER PREVENTION

In our approach to food for the body, the good news is that some common foods are blessings in disguise. Not only can we enjoy them at mealtimes, but they also can protect us against diseases, such as cancer.

The cover story of *Newsweek* (November 30, 1998) highlights food that we can eat to minimize our risk of cancer: red grapes, flaxseed, tofu, broccoli, garlic and tomatoes. A primary tumor spreads by creating new blood vessels. This growth factor can be suppressed by cox-2 inhibitors. Resveratrol is a strong antioxidant in red grapes and red wines, the yellow curry powder turmeric, rosemary and soy products can all work as cox-2 inhibitors that "...may suppress the tumor's production of growth factors" (p. 65). Flaxseed is full of omega-3 type fatty acids (also contained in fish) that "...thwart tumor growth by crowding other fats out of cells. Flaxseed may lock bad fats out of cells" (ibid.).

The use of flaxseed is not a new fad. It was popular in Mesopotamia over 4,000 years ago. Hippocrates prescribed flaxseed for intestinal discomfort. Flaxseeds are high in **lignans**, a phytoestrogen, a plant-based hormone. Not only can this be helpful in cancer prevention, but flaxseeds also help to build strong bones and a healthy heart, as well as reduce high cholesterol and triglycerides. There are two ways to use flaxseed. Each morning, we can take flaxseed oil. This should be kept in the refrigerator in a black bottle to stop the light from changing its chemical composition. We can also grind flaxseed in a coffee grinder or buy flaxseed powder and sprinkle it on bread, cereal, fruit and desserts.[10]

Tofu comes from soy beans and is packed with **genistein**, "mother nature's healing hormone."[11] In Okinawa, Japan, where tofu is the main staple, women enjoy the lowest rate of osteoporosis, breast cancer and heart disease compared to their western counterparts.

Whether well-loved or simply scorned, broccoli contains chemicals that promote the elimination of carcinogens from our cells. It seems to help in removing estrogen from the body, as well as being a rich source of antioxidants, such as **beta carotene, lutein, quercetin**, and **sulforaphane**.

Garlic, the stinking rose, can be used for numerous purposes: to lower triglycerides, cholesterol, blood pressure and reduce the risk of blood clot. It also is recommended for those suffering from diabetes and cancer. **Allyl sulfide** appears to be one of the beneficial components of garlic. Allyl sulfide forms when we cut garlic buds and then allow them to stand for 10 minutes.[12]

The ruddy complexion of tomatoes is derived from the antioxidant **lycopene**. Cooking tomatoes releases the lycopenes for absorption, transporting fat into our blood system. In a 1995 Harvard study of 48,000 men, it was found that men who ate 10 servings of tomato-enriched food weekly had approximately half the risk of prostate cancer as those who did not have the lycopenes in their diet.[13]

COOKING FOR HEALTH

The food philosopher Michio Kushi revolutionized the cooking habits of the western world. More than thirty years ago, he inspired nutritional and macrobiotic[14] studies at many institutions. The macrobiotic approach is an eclectic way of eating based on universal wisdom. It is a means to health, longevity and happiness based on common sense and age-old practices. Macrobiotics can be used in the prevention of multiple illnesses. The crux of this food-based program is the balance between dualism and monism, between yin and yang, that may help heal chronic conditions. Macrobiotics is primarily an alkaline producing diet that appears to bolster our immune system and overall health. The following composite provides a general recipe for our daily diet.

Macrobiotics recommends consuming 50-60% cooked whole grains in our daily diets, ranging from buckwheat to brown rice to barley. The grain-based protein, seitan (wheat meat or gluten) can be added and consumed several times weekly. This vegetable-based protein is becoming very popular among vegans[15] in recent times. We can find seitan in health food stores in the cooler section.

25-30% of our regular intake can be fresh, cooked vegetables: carrots, white radish (daikon), onion, burdock, brussel sprouts, Chinese cabbage, cauliflower, broccoli, kale, dandelion, mustard greens, pumpkin, and butter squash. Occasionally we can have string beans, celery, yellow squash, red cabbage, shiitake mushrooms,[16] endive, and Jerusalem artichokes.[17] Minimal use of acid producing vegetables, such as potatoes, spinach, eggplant, asparagus, zucchini and green and red peppers is recommended unless we live in a hot climate. All vegetables should be either steamed, sauteed, baked or boiled.

Soup constitutes five to ten percent of a balanced macrobiotic diet. The soup broth can be from miso or tamari sauce, naturally made and fermented from soy beans, sea vegetables and grains. Miso soup has a tremendous reputation for healing. There is a historic episode written by Shinichiro Akizuki, M.D., Medical Director of St. Francis Hospital in Nagasaki, and author of *Physical Constitution and Food.* When the U.S. bombed Nagasaki in 1945, Dr. Akizuki's hospital was a few miles from the fallout. The hospital staff and Dr. Akizuki never developed any radiation related symptoms. Dr. Akizuki attributes this protection to the miso soup they consumed daily.

We can consume another 5-10% of sea vegetables and beans. For our regular use, azuki beans, lentils and chick peas are suggested.

Soy, navy, lima and pinto beans can be consumed occasionally, as well as soy preparations, tempeh and tofu. To tempt our taste buds, try tamari sauce, sea salt and grain-based vinegar. Fruits generally are eaten cooked or naturally dried. These can serve as desserts in macrobiotics.

As civilization became increasingly mechanical, we lost our respect for the sacred power of grains. When the tomb of Tut was reopened, grains, including barley, were found among a panoply of riches and gold. In 1920, the merchants of Shanghai in China started polishing rice husks. The white color became associated with white civilization. Processed food became part of the world's cuisine, one of the cultural triggers for the rise of degenerative diseases. We now recognize that by processing a food into an unnatural form, we strip away its holistic nutritional power.

The power of whole grains literally was worshipped in many cultures. Amaranth was called "the grain of the gods" in Mexico. The Spanish conqueror, Cortez, made a rule that anyone found growing amaranth was to be beheaded. Thankfully we can still find amaranth in health food stores today. It is the richest source of protein among grains.

ENVIRONMENT-BASED EATING

A healthy diet is also based on seasonal changes, climate, and natural cycles. It is best to live in harmony with the environment, eating in accordance with seasonal and regional (locally-grown) produce. For example, tropical foods (summer fruits), such as mangos and pineapples, should be avoided during the cold season because they have a cooling effect. In winter, roots and grains should be largely consumed. In autumn, cereals, fruit, and roots are the foods-of-choice. In spring, eat sprouts. Vegetables and salads are suggested for summer time fare. It is interesting to note that the oldest healing system in the world, Ayurveda, also recommends that we live and eat in synchrony with the seasons.

Brain Food

Contemporary research is creating designer foods for the brain. According to the *Daily News, L.A. Life* (December 21, 1998) oxygen bars provide a "cure for a bad air day" (p. 3). As cities become increasingly dense, oxygen bars will become as popular as neighborhood cafes. Oxygen is food for the brain and body.

Fossil records indicate that the gingko biloba tree is the oldest tree in recorded history, being approximately 200 million years old.[18] Gingko biloba, a vasodilator, is now touted for its power to increase the flow of oxygen throughout the body and brain.

Ginseng, the elixir of life, also is a smart food. Its roots are revered as promoting eternal life. It helps in recovery from stress, building the immune system, lowering cholesterol and enhancing sexual performance.

Fatty fish (e.g., tuna, salmon and others) and walnuts are high in omega-3 fatty acids which are a good source of brain power. Seafood (oysters and fish), legumes, and whole grains are zinc-rich foods that enhance memory.

Super-Healing Foods[19]

Our unidimensional, mechanical progress is devoid of reverence for Mother Earth and literally depletes the pH balance in the soil. Our soil no longer contains the same levels of nutrients, and thus our foods have lower nutritional values. What can we do in our fast-paced society?

Personally, I recommend that we adopt a healthy balanced diet, whether we choose a diet that consists primarily of raw foods or a macrobiotic regimen. Our results indicate which diet is most suitable for our individual lifestyle, needs and constitution. I recommend regular cleansings in either case.

As consumers, we can easily be overwhelmed by the spate of new products, new research and new marketing techniques. Here are some foods that make common sense and come from God's garden. This list is meant to serve as a general reference and is not a complete list.[19]

Amla	Indian gooseberry, a high-grade food-based form of Vitamin C, the only source where the vitamin is not destroyed when cooked; tastes like rose hips.
Asparagus	Antioxidant, diuretic, anti-cancer, for kidney, swelling, rheumatoid arthritis and PMS bloating.
Banana	For ulcer, upset stomach. Elevates energy levels and moods.
Barley	For high cholesterol (an ancient heart medicine).
Bittermelon	For diabetes and blood cleansing.
Cabbage	Anti-viral, for ulcers and cataracts. Cabbage juice is anti-bacterial.[21]
Carrots	Beta carotene for eyes, heart and cancer prevention.
Celery	For high blood pressure. Diuretic, calms nerves.
Chili powder	Boosts endorphins (joy chemicals), prevents blood clots, clears congestion, causes weight reduction.

Cinnamon	Stimulates insulin production, helps after eating desserts (try at Christmas and other festivals).
Clove	For toothaches and gum problems, destroys unfriendly parasites in the stomach.
Cranberries	Diuretic, anti-viral, anti-fungal, for urinary tract infections.
Dates	Purgative, has a natural analgesic effect.
Eggplant	Reduces anxiety, lowers cholesterol, diuretic.
Fenugreek	For diabetes, ulcers, upset stomach and diarrhea (a mideast spice).
Fig	(Dried) Contains **benzaldehyde**, high in potassium and Vitamin B6, reduces tumors, for parasite, bacteria, ulcers.
Fish	For heart, cancer prevention, high blood pressure, colitis, osteoarthritis, asthma, rheumatoid arthritis, migraines and inflammatory conditions.
Garlic	Immuno-stirnulant, for cold, cough, cancer, high blood pressure and inflammation .
Ginger	For circulation, headaches, motion and morning sickness, congestion, colds, stomach pain, arthritis, cancer, diarrhea and depression.
Grapes	Antioxidant, prevents cancer, viral and bacterial infection . Grape seeds helps raise HDL (good cholesterol).
Grapefruit	Antioxidant, high vitamin C, reduces arterial blockage and high cholesterol.
Honey[22]	Soothing balm for burns, induces sleep, has a mild tranquilizing effect and antibiotic qualities.

Lemon/Lime	Vitamin C, liver detoxifier, helps prevent viral infection; also a deodorant.
Mushrooms	Shiitake, for influenza, cancer, high blood pressure and high cholesterol. Maitake,[23] for cancer, AIDS, diabetes, chronic fatigue syndrome and high blood pressure.
Nuts[24]	High in protein, fiber and vitamins, promotes HDL, antioxidant (vitamin E), for cancer and heart. **Walnuts**, brain food rich in omega-3. **Almonds**, for adrenals.[25] **Pistachios**, contain **Co Q-10** for heart.
Oats	High fiber, regulates blood sugar, for depression and curbing nicotine cravings
Olive Oil	Lowers LDL, longevity in Mediterranean regions often attributed to this.
Onion	For blood clots, bronchitis, arterial sclerosis, diabetes and hay fever. Red and yellow are rich in **quercetin**, antioxidant and anti-allergy agent
Pineapple	**Bromelain**, enzyme-rich, anti-bacterial, anti-inflammatory, for liver metabolism, blood clots, increased bone density (rich in manganese), dissolves scar tissue.
Potato (white)	High in potassium and **protease-inhibitors**, for cancer and high blood pressure.
Pumpkin seeds	For prostate, high in vitamin E and zinc
Rice	High fiber, for constipation and kidney stones.
Saffron[26]	For fever, cough, asthma, visual acuity, allergies and high blood pressure.

Seaweed and Kelp	Immunostimulant Nori, wakame and dulse are high in iodine, for thyroid and weight loss.
Turmeric	Contains **curcumin**, antioxidant, for inflammation, liver detoxification and rheumatoid arthritis.
Yogurt[27]	For bones, colds, diarrhea and upper respiratory infection.

HEALING HERBS

Herbs are like nature's laser therapy. They may help for specific conditions, and can be taken regularly as a tonic, as a prophylaxis, or as a remedy.

As we have seen, in Energy Medicine, the focus is on health versus disease. An energy-based approach primarily utilizes herbs in healing.

Astragalus [28]	For cancer patients, chronic infections and overall health
Arctic Root [29]	For increased energy, found to be more powerful than ginseng
Ashwagandha	Indian herb for vitality and sexuality
Codonopsis	For T-cell transformation and building red blood cells
Ho shou wu	For healthy hair and nails and increases fertility in both sexes
Lycium Berries	For liver regeneration, visual acuity, anemia and lung disorders
Milkthistle	For rebuilding and protecting liver cells
Schisandra	For endurance, vitality, memory, can work as a sexual tonic

| Siberian Ginseng | For endurance in athletic and/ or high altitude activities |
| St. John's Wort | For depression |

SUPER FOODS FOR COMMON AILMENTS[30]

This section can be used as supplements, along with our doctor's recommendations.[31]

Allergies	Quercetin (found in red grapes and red onion) and pycnogenol (extract of pine bark and grape seed)
Autoimmune	Turmeric (Indian herb), ginger, yucca root, glucosamine sulfate, ipriflavone (for bone density)
Cold and flu	Hot and spicy foods, ginger, echinacea, golden seal, vitamin C, inhaling steam from eucalyptus and tea tree oil; and most importantly, visualizing a time when we were deeply in love
Digestion	Pineapple, yogurt, bifidus, acidophilus, pectin (from fruit), slippery elm (herb), triphala (gentle laxative)
Energy building	Siberian ginseng, miso soup, gingko biloba, colostrum, coral calcium-rich sea salt (caution if you have high blood pressure), arctic root, ashwagandha
Female hormones	Dong quai, black cohosh, Omega-3 oil, shatavari (Indian herb)

Heart	Omega-3 oils (e.g., fish oil, flaxseed oil, extra virgin cold press olive oil), hawthorn berries, magnesium, Vitamin E, Co Q-10
Male hormones	Pygeum (from Africa), saw palmetto (prostate), zinc, ashwagandha
Sleeping	Passion flower, valerian root, kava kava, drinking warm milk

PATEL'S POWER POTIONS

Here is my personal formula for healthy living. A general rule of thumb is: eat like a king in the morning, eat like a pauper at night. Try to wake up early in the morning, and start our day with a cup of hot water with fresh lemon or lime juice. Antioxidant agents (vitamins A, C, E and selenium) can be taken twice a day; vitamins A and C in the morning, and vitamin E and selenium in the afternoon. Before leaving home, have a hearty glass of fresh carrot, ginger, beet and celery juice. Eat a wholesome cereal (devoid of artificial sweeteners) preferably with soy milk, rice milk or amazake (milk from brown rice) with bananas or berries. Multi-grain toast with cheese[32] made from tofu can be a part of our king's breakfast. Sprouts and crunchy, soaked nuts are helpful for alertness and provide a quick energy boost in the morning.

Lunch can be high in protein which helps us feel alert. I recommend yogurt, cottage cheese, bean- or grain-based protein. In the afternoon, we may feel fatigued because we hit low blood sugar levels. I recommend a green potion containing all or any of the following: wheat or barley grass, blue-green algae, chlorella, spirulina, alfalfa and green kamut. This is very helpful in boosting mid-day energy levels. In between food intervals, we can have green tea or our favorite teas.

Our evening meal can be complex carbohydrates (rice, pasta, potato) to help us to relax because they increase levels of serotonin which elevates our moods and helps us sleep soundly. A platter of our favorite fresh-cut fruits after supper will give us the essential minerals and vitamins that we need. We can sprinkle flaxseed powder, nuts, raw wheat germ and lycium berries on the fruit platter. Occasionally eating dessert makes our inner child happy. When we feel the need of an energy boost, pure royal jelly without honey can help our immune system.

FOOD FOR THE SOUL

It is said in the Old Testament "Man doth not live by bread alone."[33] We do not merely consume food by mouth, as physical matter. We also need nourishment for our soul in the form of subtle vibrations. I call this soul food. We can follow a diet based on some ideal regimen, or the newest research findings, and still we may not heal. We can exercise to exhaustion, burn calories while calculating them, and nourish ourselves with the newest nutraceuticals, and still experience difficulties in healing. I have worked with people on raw food diets or macrobiotic programs who have not achieved their desired results.

Soul food is consumed in the form of vibrations in and around us. We all have the capacity to feel these vibrations although they are not perceived through our five senses. I believe that we can benefit from periodic respites from bombardment with negative information from the media. Such vibrations are contraindicated for our health.

I recommend abstaining from eating just after an argument. Arguing triggers a basic fight-flight response that stimulates the production of hormones and chemicals throughout our bodies which are immuno-suppressants. We can go to a tree and hug it, touch a rock, take a walk, or release all our feelings by talking out loud to the clouds (beware of psychiatrists passing by). We can eat after we feel reconnected to our soul. If the above steps do not suit us, go quietly to the other person, give them a hug, and proceed to sup. This simple hug can seem difficult in the heat of the moment, but in my own experience, it works as a miraculous balm.

We also carry and create vibrations in the bedroom. Following the old adage *Never let the sun go down on your anger* retains its wisdom, and is excellent soul food.

Food is a sacred offering for the soul. When we eat, we give thanks first, "l am thankful for this wonderful food." Expressing our gratitude creates positive vibrations and elevates our mood.

I also found that surrendering to the earth provides healing vibrations. It is so simple. All we have to do is lie down on the ground and say, "I surrender to the wisdom of the universe." We can consume the ensuing peace as soul food.

Do we eat with joy? Sometimes just savoring the taste of our favorite foods can produce a flood of healing endorphins which is more beneficial than counting calories. Do we enjoy eating with someone? We can heighten our vibrations by sharing tea-for-two or splitting a popsicle with a friend. This soul food for soul mates is both efficient and economical. Instead of killing two birds with one stone,

...we can kindle two souls with one scone.

Reconciliation is instant, high-protein food for the soul. Our physical intake of food for the body will gain added medicinal properties when we are able to let go of grudges and reach out to another. It is important to note that the benefits of this soul food are not dependent on the other person's response. It is contingent upon our willingness and courage to initiate soul healing. Our awareness of enhancing positive vibrations helps us to attract more uplifting events in daily living.

If our diets contain daily soul food supplements, then eating with instinct will work in our favor. The language of our tastebuds, a wise built-in communicator, has become foreign for most of us. If our tongue indicates a taste for a t-bone, we can trust our yearning, in moderation. The delight of an ice cream cone can be the medicine-of-choice for nourishing our inner child. The crunch of popcorn may be just the thing to stimulate that smile we can share with a stranger.[34]

There is no one food in the whole world that is good for everyone all the time. The wisdom of working with *Healing Foods* is flexibility and variety. Our tongue will tell us about the taste, and our body will tell us about our needs. When we start listening to our body, we are in the realm of energy-based medicine.

The famous proverb says, "If you give a man a fish, he can eat for a day. If you teach a man to fish, he can eat for a lifetime." Learning about healing foods can yield a lifetime of good health. By listening to our own body and trusting its language we can transform our ordinary diet into food for the gods — ambrosia.

Listen to the body,
Eat with love,
And heal.

NOTES

1. In *Tales of a Shaman's Apprentice: An Ethnobotanist Searches for New Medicines in the Amazon Rain Forest* by Mark Plotkin, Ph.D.

2. Attention skiers: sprinkling a pinch of cayenne pepper in the toe of your socks prevents toes from getting cold.

3. When I visited the Santuario de Chimayo, New Mexico, the legendary healing shrine, and the American equivalent of Lourdes, I witnessed the dried red peppers hanging all over the hallowed walls.

4. Ecclesiastes 38:4

5. Stephen L. Defelice, M.D., chairperson of the Foundation for Innovation in Medicine, coined the term *nutraceutical*.

6. *The Wheatgrass Book*, 1985.

7. Dr. Otto Warburg, a Nobel laureate, discovered that cancer cells can not survive in an oxygen-rich environment. Its cell mutation occurs in oxygen-deprivation at a cellular level.

8. See https://gerson.org/gerpress/dr-max-gerson/

9. Since 1934, Norwalk (created by Dr. Norman W. Walker) is the prominent manufacturer of this custom-made juicer.

10. See Appendix for details on where to find flaxseed.

11. In *The Nutraceutical Revolution*, Richard Firshein, D.O.

12. *Newsweek* November 30, 1998, John Milner of Pennsylvania State University.

13. *op. cit.*

14. Macro, meaning long or great, and biotic, meaning life. Michio Kushi popularized this approach in the Western world . This model of nutrition emphasizes a high percentage of grain intake, as well as balanced alkaline foods.

15. Vegans are vegetarians whose diet is devoid of dairy and poultry products.

16. Shiitake is considered to be a medicinal mushroom that may be helpful for cancer patients.

17. Recent studies have confirmed that Jerusalem artichokes are helpful in controlling blood sugar levels in diabetes.

18. In *Brain Boosters: Foods & Drugs That Make You Smarter* by Beverly Potter & Sebastian Orfali.

19. Super-healing foods is a compilation of various sources for our readers. We highly recommend: Jean Carper's book *Food — Your Miracle Medicine: How Food Can Prevent and Cure Over 100 Symptoms and Problems, A Consumer's Guide to Medicines in Food: Nutraceuticals That Help Prevent and Treat Physical and Emotional Illnesses* by Ruth Winter, M.S., *Smart Guide to Healing Foods* by Katharine Colton and *Food and Healing* by Ann Marie Colbin.

20. Author makes no claims. Check with our personal physicians prior to making any dietary changes.

21. Warning: can create gastrointestinal upset and may increase migraines.

22. Honey is not advisable for infants less than one-year-old.

23. Maitake currently is available only in dry, capsule, liquid (d-fraction) forms in health food stores. Please refer to *Maitake: King of Mushrooms* by Ken Babal, C.N., and Shari Lieberman, Ph.D.

24. There is a common notion that nuts are fattening, and therefore bad, but the opposite is true. Nuts are high in friendly fatty acids.

25. I suggest soaking them overnight in water. Soaking some seeds and nuts in water may increase enzymatic activity which is very useful for various purposes, including digestion.

26. The frequent intake of saffron is associated with longevity and low rates of heart disease in Spaniards and East Indians.

27. Yogurt is considered the secret of long life in many cultures. It promotes healthy intestinal bacteria. I personally recommend fat free.

28. In some people, it may cause respiratory and abdominal distress with regular use.

29. Used in Russian space station MIR.

30. These products are available in most health food stores.

31. Two authoritative resources in this area are: *Spontaneous Healing: How To Discover and Enhance Your Body's Natural Ability to Maintain and Heal Itself* by Andrew Weil, M.D., and *The Nutraceutical Revolution*, Richard Firshein, D.O.

32. Cheese is very easy to digest. Eating low-fat cheeses in moderation according to our taste preferences is highly beneficial.

33. *Deuteronomy 8:3.*

34. In fact, eating crunchy foods helps to break the monotony of thought. When we are engaged in a lengthy task, the sound of crunchy food is helpful.

❀

CHAPTER V

HEAR AND YOUR SOUL SHALL LIVE

The Healing Power of Sound and Music

All one's life is music,
if one touches the notes rightly and in tune.

—*John Ruskin*

Sound is vibrations of energy that impact all living organisms. Music is the power of movement that enables us to transcend. We open to the possibility of healing when we listen to sound and music. There is a difference between hearing and listening. Hearing is processing stimuli through our ears; it is a physical act. **Listening** is hearing with our hearts. We heal not by hearing but by listening. The **third ear**[1] is our inner capacity to open and listen to our essence.

The shaman and the priest both have administered sound in their healing rituals since the dawn of humankind. The archeological findings of a clay five-hole ocarina, a primitive flute, indicated that music was prevalent at least 12,000 years ago. Sound was used as healing medicine.

The world is sensed as vibration, and vibration is the heart of Energy Medicine. One ripple changes the entire ocean. In this chapter, we will see the emergence of vibration in the universe, the various modalities of healing through sound, techniques for specific ailments and ways to create our own vibrational harmonics for wellness.

IN THE BEGINNING WAS SOUND

In Hebrew tradition, listening is called **shemah**. Listening is so important that it is used as the first word of the most widely-used Hebrew prayer. An entire chapter of the Old Testament is dedicated exclusively to **psalms**, "songs," as a primary means of communicating with God.

In Indian tradition, listening occurs in three phases. The first phase is **meaning**, the second is **feeling** and the third is listening with **frictionless sound**. When we hear something that creates a spark, a light that illuminates us while listening, we attribute meaning to the sound. The second phase is that meaning creates feelings in us, and these feelings create energy. The third phase occurs when our experience of meaning couples with the feeling of oneness. This transports us to a realm of **anaahat**,[2] frictionless sound. In the third phase, the duality between the listener and the sound is dissolved. The listener and the listening become one. We become that anaahat. We become a multifaceted expansion of the same, universal energy. This universal energy is called **naad brahma**, sound is God. That is, we literally can experience God by sound vibrations.

In Christianity, the origin of the world is manifested in the **Word**. *In the beginning was the word, and the word was God* (John 1:1). The world itself was created by the Word,[3] the epithet of omnipresent power.

The Greek mathematician, Pythagoras, saw that the universe was governed by the laws of music. According to Pythagoras, matter is **frozen music**. The music of the stars, the rhythm of the earth and galaxies, and all movement are vibrations of varying frequencies. We can see this cosmic dance in high-energy physics when scientists observe energy manifesting both as a wave and as a particle.

The Sufis have an extensive ritual in their mystical practices to incorporate sound, silence and movement in the realization of our true nature, our oneness with God. Sufi master, Inayat Khan, believes that music can exalt the mind above the thought of illness.

Sound For Better Or Worse

We live in a world of sound that has a profound and constant impact on us, and we can become aware of its power. It is healthy for us to surround ourselves with a life-enhancing womb of sound, the music of trees and birds, the sound of wind, the resonance of Mother Earth. There also are sounds that are detrimental to our health, like the hustling and bustling of cars and computers, the ringing of cellular phones, the buzz of beepers, the shriek of sirens and the alarm of arguments. This creates disturbances in our energy fields, and can be toxic on a long term basis.

Our Health And Sound

One day, many years ago, I was on the bus en route to downtown Los Angeles. At one stop, a tall, jovial gentleman got on the bus and sat next to me. He was humming a happy tune, so I greeted him. He told me that he had just been released from the County jail. I asked him how it felt. And he said, "Wonderful, man! The thing I was missing was the sound and the freedom of movement, people chatting, buses moving in traffic, and talking to you makes me feel that I'm alive. When I was 'in' I didn't have these sounds." This story reminds me that sometimes we are not truly grateful for what we have until it is taken away. How important it is that the sea of sound affects us and can make us well.

When man first went into space he discovered many mystical things beyond mental comprehension. One of the discoveries was an absence of earth vibrations in the spacecraft that caused nausea and a loss of bone density. This was due to the lack of gravitational pull from the earth's magnetic field, and the absence of the earth's vibrations. Mother Earth vibrates at 7.83 Hz (cycles per second). This is called the **Schumann Effect**; it is a direct current (DC) at which earth is constantly vibrating.

Modem research on human brain waves delineates four ranges of frequencies of brain waves: beta, alpha, theta and delta.[4] Alpha waves occur when we are in a state of restful awareness, and vibrate at approximately the same rate as the earth. I call this a cosmic wave. Healers move from the more hectic beta wave state into this cosmic wave to facilitate healing. It is equally important for both the healer and the healee (one who is receiving healing) to enter alpha brain wave states together. The healer, the healee and earth are all attuned to the same vibration. In my healing practice, I sometimes have seen tremendous results from dis-ease when this shift to cosmic wave happens, and chronic conditions are healed.

SOUND AND DIS-EASE

Now, we will explore two basic characteristics of sound, frequency (pitch) and amplitude (volume). Pitch is the listener's subjective perception of frequency. Amplitude, measured in decibels (dB), is the subjective perception of loudness. High decibel (dB) constant sounds have a damaging effect on living organisms, especially human beings. In the Max Planck Institute in Germany, researchers discovered that high decibel sounds have the negative effect of constricting blood vessels. Other studies suggest a correlation between high decibel sounds and a depletion of beneficial levels of minerals in the blood.

My colleague, Sir Peter Guy Manners, M.D., Ph.D., from Worcestershire, England specializes in **Cymatics**, the wave form of sound for restoring the body's natural frequencies for healing. Dis-ease, according to Dr. Manners, is characterized by the absence of certain frequencies. He uses computer-generated vibrations to treat different ailments.

At the University of California, Los Angeles, Neil Shaw and William Meecham compared a group of residents living beneath the flight pattern of the Los Angeles International Airport, and another group who lived eight miles from the airport. Shaw and Meechum discovered that the death rate was higher in those living near the airport due to chronic exposure to high dB sound levels.[5] According to Steven Halpern, Ph.D., author of *Sound Health: The Music and Sounds That Make Us Whole*, our sonic health is in danger because of the increase in the level of noise pollution.

SOUND IN NATURE

Sound vibrations influence every living thing. The range of human hearing varies[6] depending on such factors as age, diet, genetic makeup and past medical history. However, there are numerous frequencies that we do not detect with our ears that nonetheless are affecting our energy fields. For example, dolphins and dogs are able to perceive our pain through vibrations that can not be audibly detected by the human ear. Bill Schul, Ph.D., in his wonderful book entitled, *Life Song: In Harmony with All Creation*, emphasizes the human connection with all life forms.

John C. Lily, Ph.D., has conducted extensive research in the area of dolphin and human communication. Dolphins are able to imitate the vibrations of human voice and laughter at higher frequencies. Dolphins seem to empathize with humans through their sonar systems. Some facilities are discovering the therapeutic use of dolphin sound vibrations in human rehabilitation from certain maladies, such as cerebral palsy and spinal cord injuries. The Miami Dolphin Research Center is investigating further possibilities of healing utilizing dolphin therapy. I believe that disorders, such as autism and emotional withdrawal, can be helped by swimming with dolphins.

Dogs also are sensitive to human emotions. They can perceive our emotions and pathological states via sound and smell vibrations. In my experience, dogs can perceive and gauge our mood variations via sound. Human language becomes accessible to dogs not via the alphabet but by the vibrations we produce. Man's best friend is also a gift to humankind, especially for our long life as we have seen in Chapter III.

Music differentially affects plants. Tests conducted by Dorothy Retallack on morning glories showed that when popular rock music was played, the plants turned away from the music source and literally withered. When baroque and classical music were played, the plants were bouncing with health. In an interview with *The Denver Post*, Ms. Retallack reported that daily listening to soft music for three weeks caused plants to flourish. When exposed to the melodies of Bach, plants leaned 35 degrees toward the music source. Her fascinating book *The Sound of Music and Plants* is full of amazing insights. The subtle sound vibrations, even those beyond human range, have a tremendous effect on our communication with nature.[7]

SOUND APPLICATION AND BENEFITS[9]

Music has a significant impact on human beings, as well as plants. Several practical resources for everyday use are highlighted here. To enhance alpha brain wave activity, I find that Paul Horn's *Inside the Great Pyramid**[8] is highly effective.[9] His audiotape series are recorded at various power centers (e.g., the Taj Mahal). Rik Ved's *Ninth and Tenth Mandal** are effective in releasing past cellular memories. These ancient incantations are performed in Sanskrit. Although we may not understand the words, they can be a great tool for transformation because they work at the level of our analog system. *Gregorian Chants**, Monastic Choir of the Abbey of St. Peter of Solesmes, especially the *Midnight Mass and Mass of the Day* directed by Dom Jean Claire in western France, can be energizing and healing. I recommend them in

Latin for the same reason stated above. Our hearts can hear what our minds cannot understand, but if given a chance, our cerebral minds can interfere in the healing process.

In order to induce spirit, I recommend the unique field recordings by Smithsonian/Folkways Records *Tuva: Voices from the Center of Asia** that contains melodic patterns created by shamans in their sacred communications with the Divine. I personally find that morning is most congenial for bringing shamanistic energies. Lighting a candle before playing sacred music will accentuate the mood and enhance healing.

Philip Halboth, Ph.D., and Lloyd Glauberman, Ph.D., created a tape called *Hypno-Peripheral Processing**. The recording is done in a story-telling format where two people speak simultaneously to both sides of our brain; the left side of our brain being logical and sequential, and the right brain being creative and nontemporal. Listening to two stories at the same time can help us to surpass limiting thresholds and open us to possibilities. The *H PLUS** series by the Monroe Institute has far-reaching effects on changing human thought and behavior patterns.

Steven Halpern's *Audio Active* subliminal series* *Sound Sleep, Overcoming Substance Abuse, Recovering from Alcoholism* and *Peak Performance* are effective resources for changing behavior patterns.

Lawrence Katz creates shamanistic healing sounds that accelerate self-healing. His use of sound with electromagnetic tools and crystals helps us to become whole.

Cecilia's *Amazing Grace: Prayer to the Whales*, always transports me to a heightened state of healing.

Sharyn Scott's collection of songs and lyrics spontaneously opens the door to the soul. It moves me, and brings tears to my eyes every time I listen. If we want to feel the presence of Spirit, listen to the voice of this angel.

Healthy Pleasures, by Robert Ornstein, Ph.D., and David Sobel, M.D., elegantly describes various examples of how music can work as medicine. For example, studies have found that soothing music has a valium-like effect. If someone is suffering from acute heart or other problems, the soothing effect of music may help, in addition to other medical interventions. Patients may benefit from sound therapy before, during and after surgical procedures. In a study conducted at the University of California, Davis, Medical Center, positive verbal instructions coupled with music helped patients throughout all phases of surgery.[10]

In a study on premature babies, Brahms' lullaby correlated with weight gain, a critical factor in survival. Babies gained weight more quickly, and were discharged earlier from the hospital. I recommend the lullaby cure even for adult babies like us to help calm our restless minds. With crying infants, the audiotape series *Baby-Go To-Sleep** has been used in more than 4,000 medical facilities. These tapes can be used at home to facilitate sleep with infants.

We have seen the practical implications in adults and infants. Have we ever considered music therapy for plants? Dan Carlson's Scientific Enterprises has created *Sonic Bloom,* a program for boosting the blossom potential of our favorite begonia and enhancing our green thumbs. This includes an audiotape and a spray supplement.

SOUND HEALING TIME

Everything has a time and a rhythm. Modem science is beginning to acknowledge and incorporate **chronobiology**, chrono, meaning time and bio, meaning life, in medical practices. In the ancient Jndian *Vedas,* there is a concept called **pahar**, where different moments have different connotations based on their synchronicity with cosmic vibrations. For example, chanting, singing or listening to certain melodic rhythms called **ragas** at different times (pahar) affect us differently.

I recommend the following guidelines for beginning practice with a few ragas: **bhairavi** (early morning), **kalavati** (midnight), **yaman** (early evening) and **malkauns** (evening). The vibration of the morning ragas are revitalizing, the afternoon ragas are energizing, and the evening ragas are deeply relaxing.

Pahar And Vibration Of The Organs

The organs of our body have stored vibrations from the past. For eons vibrations have been metabolized in our cells, and stored in our major organs and DNA as cellular memories. Many different techniques can be used to release these "sick vibrations," such as Qigong, reiki, tai chi, meditation, yoga, affirmations and therapeutic touch. There also is a pahar, an optimal time, to release these cellular memories. In this interim, we can heal the specific organ and specific emotion (as discussed in Chapter II). Following is the pahar-organ-emotion continuum:

>   mid morning: spleen – worrying
>   mid-day: heart – extreme emotion
>   early afternoon: liver – anger
>   late afternoon: lung – sadness
>   early evening: kidney – fear

During the first phase of pahar, we lie down and surrender to spirit. While doing the pahar-organ-emotion continuum, we visualize positive, complementary emotions. For example, we project images of serenity and acceptance when concentrating on healing our liver, freedom for the spleen, courage and strength for kidney, joy for the lung, and balance and harmony for the heart.

In the second phase, after releasing past vibrations and replacing them with new energies, we are ready to begin using harmonics for healing. We prepare by centering ourselves in silence and practicing deep breathing. When we feel a sense of oneness, we begin to make sounds in smooth, flowing, even tones, according to the following chart:

Organ	Sound
liver	shoe
heart	hoe
spleen	who
lungs	sea
kidneys	crow

Using harmonics and practicing with belief will bring remarkable results. This practice was one of the techniques that helped me to heal from a supposedly incurable dis-ease.

OUR VOICE AS A KEY

Jeffrey Thompson, D.C.,[13] Director of the Center for Neuroacoustic Research, has developed a technique called **bio-tuning**. Bio-tuning is based on the premise that our body is a composite of energy or vibrational patterns. Dr. Thompson uses a series of sophisticated tests to locate energy imbalances in different body systems. For example, he utilizes an acupuncture meridian identification (AMI) device, a computer-based machine that measures chi energy in the body's meridians.

A **sound treatment** is then developed according to the individual's unique quantum pattern, based on identifying a single frequency that causes a global body balance. Like creating sound on a wine glass, we can discover the perfect frequency that causes an individual's body cells to resonate. The individual's voice is then digitally-processed via computer, and is reproduced at various octaves to induce healing at different levels of energy within the body. Dr. Thompson describes achieving outstanding and lasting results using bio-tuning.

Sound Initiation

There are other ways to access healing using sound techniques, such as organ-specific sounds for healing.[14] During meditation, the ancient Rishis identified particular sound vibrations associated with healing specific organs. These insights have been handed down through the ages by oral tradition during the initiation process. Such sound healing practices still are used in yoga and Qigong today.

We can always utilize our own sound even if we do not listen to audio tapes or undergo sophisticated initiations.[15] All vowels in the English language vibrate with a quality that can impact our major energy centers in a healing fashion. We can use the basic vowel sounds **I-E-A-O-U** and our own voice to initiate healing. The following chart delineates the vowels that are affiliated with certain energy centers in the body. Producing these sounds helps heal energy imbalances in the organ manifesting dis-ease:

Vowel	Region
ee	brain
ay	throat
ah	heart
oh	stomach
uu	lower pelvic

Sound	Condition to heal
iiiiiiiiiii…	Sinus congestion, cold, migraine headache
eeeeeeee…	Sore throat, thyroid malfunction
ahhhhh…	Heart conditions, allergies, lung congestion, asthma
ohhhhh…	Lethargy, circulatory problems, digestive disorders
youuuuu…	Menstrual cramps, prostate problems, sexual dysfunction

PRANIC HARMONIC HEALING

We can apply sound practices in sustaining and promoting our general health. **Harmonics** are concurrent vibrations of parts of the whole. The human voice may appear to be a single, simple vibration, but it actually is a composite vibration enriched with timbre, resonance and overtones. Quite literally, we can use our own voices as healing instruments that alter the vibrations of our cells.

Before we begin, we need to prepare ourselves for optimal reception of harmonic therapy. We literally intake **prana**, life force, by breathing. **Pranayama**, the ancient Indian science of breathing, is affiliated with a long and healthy life. In our restless world, we have become shallow, mechanical breathers; we tend to breathe superficially from our chest.

In pranic breathing, placing one hand on our stomach may gently shift us to breath deeply from our diaphragms, feeling our abdomens expand as we consciously receive prana.[16] After deep breathing for at least two minutes, or until we feel relaxed, we are ready to begin applying healing harmonics to our cells.

Moving our hand from our stomach to our nose, we begin to practice alternating nostril breathing. We begin by softly closing one nostril with our middle finger as we inhale, and then hold our breath for a count of 5-10 seconds (whatever is most comfortable depending on our medical condition, weight, age, etc.). Pressing the thumb against the other nostril and exhaling, we then take our next inhalation through that same nostril. Continue alternating the entire cycle three times.

We start by creating an elongated yawning sound, allowing our jaws to relax and fully release, while saying ahhhh. After this cathartic process, the next sound we begin to produce is the sound of our **authentic voice**, similar to our voices just after we wake up.

Unwittingly, since birth, our voices integrate and carry distortions of past emotional traumas. Past criticisms, carpings and complaints unconsciously create an armor that shields and distorts our voices. This armor actually blocks us from reaching our healing potential because it interferes with our ability to connect with our authentic voices.

After reclaiming our real selves, inhale fully, and then create the stretched vibration, **aumm**...[17] as we exhale. The longer we can extend this sound, the more healing resonance is generated. This primordial seed sound can balance the energy systems throughout the entire body.

THE TOMATIS METHOD[18]

The French physician Alfred Tomatis, M.D., can truly be called the Michelangelo of sound for health. Dr. Tomatis discovered that our voices can create what our ears can hear. That is, we can not resonate with multi dimensional sound unless we can hear a broad spectrum. According to *Vogue* (British), June, 1992, Tomatis discovered a collective ethnic "ear," a society's spectrum of hearing based on their preferred frequencies. Americans hear between 750-3,000 Hz, Germans hear 100- 3,000 Hz, English 2,000-12,000 Hz, and French 1,000-2,000 Hz.

Dr. Tomatis also found that high frequency vibrations are energizing. Gregorian chants, where monks sing in unison, contain high frequency vibrations (up to 2,000- 4,000 Hz) that are processed by the central nervous system and then are distributed throughout the body as energizing electrical impulses.

Dr. Tomatis prescribes Mozart, and not any other composer. In his opinion, "Chopin tends to encourage day-dreaming and absent-mindedness linked to learning disabilities; Beethoven can deepen feelings of depression and melancholic withdrawal; while Paganini, Wagner or military marches may over-arouse children to irritability, aggression and hyperactivity."[19]

In my seminars, by listening to an individual's sound patterns, I can detect in which area of the body they are experiencing depleted energy. I then produce harmonics with my voice that restore the energy balance for the needed area.

SACRED SOUND

All over the world, there are **mantras**, sound meditations, that have the power to shift our destiny toward the desired direction. In different traditions, mantras and hymns have been passed down through the ages for energizing our potential and preserving rituals.

I received a powerful mantra during my initiation in the holy Tibetan cave of Padmasambhava. I want to share this rare mantra for the good of all, requesting that it be used in that spirit:

Om ah hum vajra guru paymeh Siddhi hum

ॐ अहं ह्वज्र गुरु पय्मेः सिद्धिहि

In the ancient Aramaic language, Jesus called God, our Divine Father-Mother, by the beautiful mantra:

Abwoon[20]

The heart-felt Greek phrase, meaning "Lord, hear our prayer," can be adopted as a personal mantra:

Kyrie eleison

In Hebrew, calling upon the mystical power *ehyeh asher ehyeh* "I Am That I Am," designates that a spark of God resides in each one of us.

אהיה אשר אהיה

Lakota elder and shaman Wallace Black Elk wrote a sacred prayer for me that blesses all our relationships:

Mitakuye Oyas'in Wanbli cik'ala.

Sound of Silence

We can center ourselves in silence without judgment to feel the presence of Spirit in everyday life. We can enter into the choiceless awareness of silence by witnessing existing sound. Silence can become a healing meditation that we can perform any time we like. This sound break of witnessing silence will replenish our entire energy system. My friend, Mickey Hargitay, a former Mr. Universe (1955) and who played the legendary Hercules in the movies, one day shared with me,"I have the sound here (touching his hand to his heart), and I listen to it all the time, and that is my music."

A seeker of Zen went to China. Upon his return to the imperial court of Japan, the emperor asked him, "What did you learn, Kakua?" Kakua pulled a flute from his robe, played a single note, bowed down and left the room. God is as simple as one note of the flute. Beauty can be felt in a single note, as well as in a symphony. God is everywhere, in silence and in sound...

Listen and heal.

EXERCISES FOR TRANSFORMATION AND HEALING

1. **Flowing Water**: Bring flowing water, like a fountain, into our lives. The sound of flowing water will help energize us. An audio tape of some form of running water can be an alternative.

2. **Joyful noises**: In our hectic, daily routines, we can make senseless, joyful noises in between our scheduled activities. For example, we can whistle or hum our favorite tunes. This can be mood-enhancing and add to our happiness.

3. **Harmonics in the Shower**: Our bathtubs and showers can be our hub of healing. We can rejuvenate by creating harmonics under the showerhead or immersed in a soothing tub.

4. **Environmental Echoes**: Many of us have become alienated from nature in our modern lives. Listening to the sounds of nature, thunder, rain, rustling leaves, a stream, birds singing, crickets chirping, can be synchronizing for our cells and restorative for our soul. Environmental audio tapes or CD's can be used as accessible and relatively inexpensive resources.

5. **Good vibrations**: Sharing time with those we love is good medicine. We may receive an added power boost by listening frequently to the sound of someone's voice that is particularly appealing to our cells and selves .

NOTES

1. See *The Third Ear* by Joachim-Ernst Berendt.

2. A. Friction Sound   B. Frictionless Sound

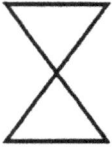

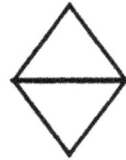

    In a confrontational relationship the singular point of contact results in disharmony (A). When the triangle's points do not confront each other they become harmonious (B)

3. It is interesting to note that in many other ancient scriptures, such as Egyptian and Sumarian, this same analogy of creation can be found stemming from a sacred word.

4. Beta are normal, active, waking-state brain waves. We experience theta and delta waves in deep sleep, trance and deep meditation.

5. In *Science News*,1983, *Airport Noise Linked with Heart Disease.*

6. Found in Jonathan Goldman's pioneering work in the authoritative book, *Healing Sounds: The Power of Harmonics.*

7. For further details refer to Dr. Schul's *Life Song: In Harmony with all creation.*

8. Audiotapes followed by an asterisk are not to be used while driving or operating machinery.

9. This recording was sacredly produced. Paul Horn asked permission to shut off all fluorescent lighting in the King's Chamber to ensure that the Pyramid's natural magnetic field was undisturbed.

10. The effect of music was comparable to a 2.5 milligram intravenous dose of valium.

11. Please refer to the masterful work *The Secrets Our Body Clocks Reveal: How to Tune into Your Body's Rhythms to Perform at Your Peak Day or Nigh*t written by Susan Perry and Jim Dawson.

12. These sound vibrations were revealed in higher states of meditation.

13. This section is based on a telephone interview with Dr. Thompson.

14. Kenneth Cohen, *The Way of Qigong: The Art and Science of Chinese Energy Healing*, reviews the sound-organ pairings.

15. These techniques are intended to be complimentary to, and practiced in conjunction with, other allopathic treatments. Author makes no medical claim.

16. It is interesting to note that, when I do healing, people who tend to have difficulties receiving rarely use the proper technique of diaphramatic breathing. The sound specialist Dennis Rodgers recommends moving the tongue back slightly to create a vortex of air that swirls up and through the sinuses when practicing pranic breathing.

17. **Aum** is an ancient Sanskrit mantra to vibrate and align our energy patterns with our Source.

18. Dr. Tomatis has established international treatment centers. A client listens through a machine called an **electronic ear,** mainly to the voice of their mother and Mozart. The electronic ear eliminates middle-frequency vibrations, and the listener hears only high-frequency sounds for many sessions in promoting health.

19. *Vogue* (British) June, 1992, p. 170.

20. Neil Douglas-Klotz, *Blessings of the Cosmos.*

CHAPTER VI

EARTH MEDICINE

Biology of Environment

Everything in Nature contains
all the powers of Nature.
Everything is made of one hidden stuff.

— Emerson

Mind body marriage can create healing vibrations for our health, as we have reviewed in previous chapters. We have learned different techniques for self-healing. We will now integrate the unique effects of environment into our panoramic approach. There is a constant, dynamic interchange between us and our environment. When we realize we have a great degree of control over our environment, we can make conscious choices that tailor our surroundings to promote our wellbeing.

Mainstream medical practices have focused little attention on the ways in which our environment can enhance our health. In many European countries, such as Germany, **bau-biologie**, biology of the environment, has been prescribed as popular medicine.

In the following chapter, we will explore the relationship between **Earth Medicine** and the history of humankind. We then will investigate the deleterious effects of two types of pollution, geopathic (earth-generated) and electromagnetic (human-made). Lastly, we will address the resolution of pollution, ways in which we can create our own healing environments.

EARTH MEDICINE AND CULTURE

In India, based on reverence for nature's inherent spirit, an art called **vastukala**, the art of creating harmony in our habitat, was practiced widely.[1] The sacred art of vastukala was handed down from generation to generation. A sense of environmental conscience was evident In India as early as the third century B.C. Historical records indicate that the emperor Ashoka banned adulterating drinking water and pillaging forests. This royal declaration was carved into stones, and its relics can be found in Indian museums today. Ashoka's compassionate view of nature continues to touch my heart, especially as I see events unfolding in our modem world.[2]

In ancient Greece, Earth Medicine was practiced under **genius loci**, the spirit of the location. Earth was conceptualized and treated as a living organism. The temple of Delphi was devoted to **Gaia**, the goddess of earth.

Under the Islamic influence in Africa, China and Madagascar, Earth Medicine was practiced as **vintana**. In vintana, a sense of sacredness was created in the home and at burial sites.

In China in 2,000 B.C., the emperor Yu cited the use of dowsing rods in the first book on dowsing. **Dowsing** is the ancient art used to discover underground water and sacred places, such as construction sites for building temples.[3] Today, dowsing has many other uses.

In modem Western civilization, reverence for Mother Earth, and finding healthy and congenial sites, was practiced as **geomancy**.[4] Geomancy is the art of finding the optimum place on the landscape in which to locate sacred places of transformation, such as hospitals, homes, churches and institutes of higher learning. Since transformation can occur at different levels — physical, spiritual, and emotional — it is important to find the optimal location, that place that is in harmony with its intended purpose. D.H. Lawrence beautifully illustrates this,

"Different places on the face of the earth have different vital effluence, different vibration, different chemical exhalation, different polarity with different stars: call it what you like, but the spirit of place is a great reality."[5]

We can see that elements of the earth vibrations, locations, and sanctity, were respected in many cultures. This is what I call Earth Medicine. As our civilization became industrialized, the power of places and our planet per se lost their esteemed positions. Archeologist and aromatic consultant John Steele describes our contemporary alienation from our relationship with the earth, calling it **geomantic amnesia**. Steele says that we have lost our memory of whole systems.[6] We have become disconnected from the natural rhythms of the earth. We have lost our footing in the cosmological dance. For example, the vast networks of urban artificial lighting make our relationship with the stars dysfunctional. Practicing geomancy enables us to gain the greatest energies from the earth rather than building randomly and unconsciously in places that induce negative effects.

In the planetary shift we are experiencing that our consciousness is expanding and we are reuniting with our reverence for earth. The modem popularity of **feng shui**[7] reflects this trend. Feng shui provides practical ways of rearranging our environment to promote health and wealth. Feng shui emphasizes spatial arrangements, color and natural elements in its approach.

Dowsing For Energies

Dowsing can be used for purposes other than locating water and sacred sites. It also can be utilized to detect energy fluctuations within the human body, locate lost animals, find lost objects, determine optimal food-body type combinations or to find resolutions. It can be done in person or long-distance.

Many times individuals call me from different areas of the country to assist them with health and interpersonal issues. Utilizing diverse methods of dowsing, in many instances I have been able to indicate energy imbalances in the body prior to any formal medical intervention. In my experience, negative energy states can be sensed prior to manifestation in the bodymind as dis-ease. I believe the balance of energies can be restored early on before they manifest as symptoms.

In my healing journey, I became aware of Earth Medicine in 1991 at a conference I was attending in Pasadena, California. Richard Gerber, M.D., author and presenter on *Vibrational Medicine*, introduced me to Vince Wiberg, a dowser. He warmly encouraged me to experience his dowsing skills.

After the conference that evening, Wiberg came to my home to share and teach his dowsing techniques. He first dowsed my body. Although he had no knowledge of my past medical history, he marked the low bioenergetic points on my body at the same place where I had had my surgery. I was spellbound.

I believed in the power of dowsing energies from that moment forth. I suddenly became aware of tingling, heat sensations in my hands. My face changed. He saw my face, and he handed me two L-shaped copper rods. I picked them up and spontaneously went through the energy system in his body, just as he had done on me. As I went through Wiberg's energy scan, I indicated lower and higher energy points on his body. He was smiling and nodding his head.

Wiberg later confirmed that, although I was a novice, my natural dowsing skill was accurate. For example, when I dowsed his hands, I sensed low energy vibrations; Wiberg confirmed that he had arthritis which troubled his fingers. I have used dowsing rods in my healing practice since that time.

Wiberg shared an interesting story with me. He hired a service to cut down two trees in his yard. A few weeks later, I phoned him. I was surprised to discover that he had a massive heart attack. Wiberg attributed this to his lack of compassion. As a dowser, and a believer in the sacredness of energy in all life forms, he reported that he forgot to ask the permission of the trees before having them cut down.

A note for healers: I learned from this experience about the relative wisdom of deed, need and greed. Whenever we use techniques to interact with energy, we must do it with goodness in our hearts. Not from our need, but based on our compassion for other people's needs. These skills are gifts and must be used for the goodness of humankind and not for personal gain. Every time we use dowsing or other tools of energy reading, it is acceptable to receive a fee for our services but the healee should determine the final fee. We must remember the purpose of all the sacred healing arts is to help others and to do so with compassion.

GEOPATHIC ZONES AND DIS-EASES

Geo means earth and **pathic** means disease-creating. Both the earth and organisms are composed of vibrations. The effects of negative energies manifest when there are disturbances in the energy fields. There is a wide body of research that points to the relationship between dis-ease and the earth's currents. Gustav von Pohl described this in his pioneering work, *Earth Currents: Causative Factor of Cancer and Other Diseases*. World renowned researcher and oncologist Hans Nieper, M.D. found that the vast majority of his cancer patients lived in high geopathic zones.[8] In *Earth Radiation*, Kathe Bachler depicts the correlation between negative earth energies and many dis-eases, such as allergies, arthritis and cancer. Bachler's book contains startling discoveries based on the author's experience dowsing more than 3,000 homes in more than 14 countries.

Many things can create harmful earth rays. For example, homes, especially sleeping areas, that are located over underground water, cracks in the earth, mineral deposits, gamma rays, and damp ceilings create hot spots (geopathic disturbances). The moral of the story is that it appears best to sleep high and dry.

DOWSING DELIVERS

In my dowsing practice, I have found that when we chronically feel restless or have a hard time falling asleep, it can be helpful to bring a professional dowser to check the telluric radiation (earth rays) in the bedroom. If we are experiencing repeated symptoms, such as sneezing, coughing, migraine headaches, or joint pain, in a particular area in our home, it tends to reflect energy imbalances. If I discovered that I had a major illness, I would not sleep in the same location again.

For those of us who do not have access to a personal dowser, I have a solution. I suggest bringing a cat and a dog into our bedroom with the furniture removed. Without interfering, we can observe where they sit and cuddle up. Dogs sit in areas that are beneficial to humans whereas cats gravitate to zones of geopathic disturbance. Insects also thrive on negative earth energies. When renting or buying a home, avoid "creepy" places that have beehives on the property or ants crawling inside the house.

If we already live in a place that has a hot spot and we are not able to move, I have found from my practice that placing a blue omega on the hot spot may neutralize negative energies for a while. Coil a piece of copper wire (approximately 1/8 inch wide), and bend it into a 6 x 6 inch shape of an omega Ω the last letter of the Greek alphabet. Using cellophane tape, attach it to a piece of blue cardboard. It is advisable to replace our blue omega every several months because the apparatus loses its potency from constant earth currents.

SOIL VIBRATIONS

The French engineer and genius Georges Lakhovsky,[9] author of the classic work *The Secret of Life: Cosmic Rays and Radiations of Living Beings*, unearthed a correlation between the quality of the soil and the distribution of dis-ease. In various areas of Paris, soil having high levels of sand and limestone were found to correlate with lower rates of cancer; soil high in plastic clay had significantly higher cancer rates. Sandstone, gravel, limestone and primitive rocks seem to function as insulators, absorbing cosmic vibrations. This seems to be beneficial for health, according to Lakhovsky. Soil with clay, mineral deposits and slate appear to serve as electrical conductors that can increase the spread of telluric radiation.

The relationship between food and soil is inseparable. The contemporary trend of organically-grown foods reflects an expanding consciousness about the earth and our health. Organically-grown foods are raised in soils free of unnatural chemicals which can be harmful to normal cell function. Many of us cannot afford the complete spectrum of organically-grown foods for our regular diets, so for our daily consumption, I suggest we try to buy organic fruits and vegetables whose skins we consume, such as grapes, strawberries, apples and peaches.

SOMETHING IN THE AIR

Our moods, chemical balance sense of well-being and aggressivity can be affected to large extent by the ions in the air. Ions can have either positive or negative electrical charges. Several studies indicate that when high concentrations of positively charged ions are in the air, crime, casualties and mental restlessness increase.[10]

Ionic imbalances in the air have different names in different areas of the world: in Israel, it is **sharav**; **sirocco** in Italy; **mistral** in France;

foehn in Switzerland and Germany; **purobia haava** in India; and **Santa Ana** in California. All these air-born ionic imbalances cause a dance of disharmony in human behavior patterns.

We can do several things to bridge the imbalance and bring in negatively charged ions. We can install a reliable negative charge ionizer. Nature also provides alternatives. Going to the mountains, the sea and places near running water (especially waterfalls), are beneficial because of the negative currents being conducted in these areas. Do we remember the feeling of dancing in the rain? The reason for this is that drizzling rain changes the ionic imbalance and brings harmony, causing an elevation in mood. As Longfellow elegantly said, "Back to their springs, like the rain, shall fill them full of refreshment."[11]

Indoor carpeting, synthetic clothing, asphalt, plastic surfaces and concrete also create ionic imbalances. Modem urban architecture tends to desecrate nature's inherent healing powers. The famous architect Frank Lloyd Wright joked about being able to design a house that could bring about a divorce within six months. With his structural knowledge, he designed creations that were woven in harmony with nature's rhapsody.

Walking barefoot on the grass may help us to diffuse static electricity and toxic vibrations created by treading on synthetic fibers. We can also wear natural fabrics, such as cotton, wool and silk. Removing carpeting and refurbishing hardwood floors can help reduce allergy symptoms since molds, bacteria, and mildew tend to grow in carpeting. Using organic cleansing substances, such as natural bee's wax wood polishes and natural detergents, creates a healthier milieu. As mentioned in previous chapters, inviting Mother Nature to come inside also promotes harmony, such as having an indoor fountain and potted plants.

Hazardous elements, such as radon gas and lead, can be detrimental to our health.[12] Radon gas, a radioactive substance exuding from some soils, may be linked to lung cancer. If we live in an old home that has lead-based paints and old plumbing fixtures, it is advisable to check to ensure against exposure to toxic levels. Especially in children, chronic exposure to lead is associated with neurological deficits, hyperactivity and developmental delays.

HUMAN-MADE POLLUTION

Our human cells have never been exposed to such a buzzing of electromagnetic energies as they are today. In modern society, more and more artificial energies create radiation fields that relentlessly bombard our body's cellular system. Many researchers worldwide are warning us about electrical and electromagnetic pollution in regards to our health and dis-ease. Nancy Wertheimer brought this awareness to the public eye in 1979. She reported that children living around heavy power lines had twice the rate of cancer found in children not exposed to this pollution. Dr. David Savitz of the University of North Carolina reported that 20% of childhood cancer appears to be related to exposure to high electromagnetic fields (>3 milligauss[13]). In another study by Dr. Marilyn Goldhaber and a team of researchers at Kaiser Permanente Health Group in California, pregnant women who were working with computers for more than 20 hours weekly were found to have twice the rate of miscarriage as workers not so exposed.[14]

We may want to rethink our common practice of using electric blankets and heated water beds. Sleeping directly next to artificial sources of electricity may create disturbances in magnetic fields. It has been correlated with decreased levels of melatonin production.

We may want to reevaluate our use of quick-fix microwave ovens. Some studies indicate the frequencies used for heating foods in microwaves may alter human blood chemistry levels, such as reducing hemoglobin levels and causing short-term decreases in lymphocytes.[15]

The epidemic use of cellular phones is receiving close monitoring. Preliminary studies seem to demonstrate correlations between cellular phone use and physical changes. Let us note that, "the FDA has issued an advisory warning that hand-held cellular phones should be used only when necessary..."[16]

POLLUTION PREVENTION

Consumer attention is being drawn to numerous contradictory studies emerging in the media and in scientific journals. We can easily become confused about what choices to make in our world of mass microwave radiation. I believe in prudent avoidance. In one example, the *Boston Globe* instructed its employees to move their desks at least three feet away from video display terminals.[17]

I follow the dictum of Dr. Robert Becker, twice nominated for the Nobel Prize, "I advocate a maximum field strength of 1 milligauss for continuous exposure to 60-Hz fields."[18] I have sampled various electromagnetic testing meters to survey electromagnetic fields in residential and commercial areas. I found that the TriField meter was most user-friendly. By finding the ambience, the existing magnetic field, we can become aware of the conditions in which we live, and follow Dr. Becker's advice by moving away from sources that generate more than 1 mG. The source of electricity may be coming from televisions, computers, stereos, radios, alarm clocks, answering machines, hair dryers and electric kitchen appliances. We can create a serene environment by removing all electrical paraphernalia, at least in our bedroom, especially any that are near our head.

To my knowledge, there is nothing available for consumers that completely blocks magnetic fields.[19] Before renting or buying a home, we can consider checking the ambience. I carry the TriField Meter for this purpose. I also conduct this testing for others, upon request.

Plants may provide a buffer against harmful electromagnetic influences, especially shrubs and conifers. Roger Coghill, author of *Electro Pollution: How to Protect Yourself Against It*, mentions the Cypressus Leylandii and Cereus Peruvianus cactus. Spider plants and Boston ferns, to name a few, may have potential protective benefits indoors.

Rita Holgers Awana, D.N., Ph.D., author of *Radiation: The Hidden Enemy*, discovered several things that might be helpful in diffusing the negative energies. According to the author, Garrett Snuff can be kept alongside sources of negative energy, like video display terminals (VDT). She discovered that rubies and pearls may have a positive effect in stimulating the body with no adverse effects.

Diodes can be used to help us protect our bodies against low-level radiations. They can be carried in a pocket, worn as jewelry or placed in our sleeping area.

SICK BUILDING SYMPTOMS

Do we have itchy skin, red eyes, sinus congestion or a depressed feeling in a specific location? Perhaps in a home or office? Our instincts may be working to protect us. Past vibrations left by a previous occupant may be condensed in that area and may be registering on our subtle senses. Fungus, mold and bacteria deposited in the static air cannot be seen by our eyes yet can be felt by a sensitive person.

Pheromones convey emotions, both positive and negative. For example, residue from anger can condense in a location in the form of pheromones. The next time we feel depressed or sick in certain places, we may be picking up pheromones left by another person. If we are working in such a place from 9:00-5:00, what shall we do?

REBUILDING BALANCE

We can cleanse our energy field of the residue of previous energy vibrations. One way of doing this is by taking a eucalyptus bath any time we feel negative. Eucalyptus is an energizing essential oil. Using 4-5 drops in the bathtub or putting them on our shoulders before taking a shower can be beneficial. Eucalyptus is an eye irritant, so we must be careful not to touch our eyes when handling it. After bathing, we can cleanse our vibrational fields by burning white sage. Native Americans have used white sage for generations to evaporate negative energies.

If we have an argument, personal conflict, or experience separation (even the loss of a pet), sprinkle rice in four corners of the room. Begin in the bedroom, even if the turmoil did not occur there. Start in the eastern corner, and proceed clockwise. Burning cypress oil also helps to cleanse painful vibrations.

At work, sick office symptoms can be helped by using tea tree oil in a diffuser. This is especially helpful when symptoms are generated by fungus, mold and bacteria, indicated by a preponderance of cold and allergy symptoms. If vibrations are of anger and hostility, diffusing rose oil can neutralize them. If it is an agitated environment, soothing can be created by lavender oil. After a long weekend, the smell of grapefruit and rosemary oils help to regain our work momentum and beat the Monday blues. Citrus smells, such as lemon, are most useful when working with word processors and computers. One study has indicated that errors can be reduced by 54%.[20]

When we confront a hostile situation at work, we can deflect negative energies by other practical remedies. I use feng shui unfailingly for this purpose.[21] We should check with our supervisor prior to implementing any of the following suggestions. Placing a flower vase on our table, bringing water in a clear container or setting up a miniature fountain or a crystal can ground negative energies.

I am including only a few specific cures of feng shui. The head of the bed should face the entranceway; it should not be within the line of entry but set aside as if to create an open passage when we enter the room. Sleeping in direct line with the entranceway creates hectic energies in the bedroom. Sleeping under beams and columns may block the energies in body organs beneath those structures. If our ceilings are constructed in that fashion, then we can put a pair of flutes with red tassels hanging on them, with the mouthpieces pointing upward and tilting toward each other.

The entrance to our residence should be bright and cheerful. If it is a narrow passage, which can create a sense of discouragement, we can balance that by putting mirrors on both sides, and keeping a bright, welcoming light on. Hanging wind chimes and crystals near the windows and doors can bring new energies in our life. If our residence is overpowered by taller, neighboring buildings, which can symbolically hamper our progress, we can deflect that by sticking a mirror outside facing that building to deflect its energy back to itself. Putting green and wooden decorations in the east corner of our bedroom may symbolically help in our health condition. Placing a fountain in the north side may help boost our careers.

Balancing With Color

Colors have a tremendous impact on our moods and metabolism. We can enhance our energies and increase our creative output by changing colors. Peach and pink colors can be comforting and imaginative. Green can be nurturing and inspire new growth. Blue tends to be calming. If we are lethargic, red can boost our energy levels. Red can also heighten male sexual energies. Violet appears to be an aphrodisiac for women. Yellow and orange can be energizing. With their pristine natures, white and beige can be uplifting. It is always enjoyable to restore our intuitive sense and analyze our color patterns in terms of seasons. For example, olive-skinned individuals have a proclivity for celebrating autumn colors. For this person, using earth tones may create balance and harmony.

PRACTICAL EARTH MAGIC

Magic is everywhere. All we need to do is expand our awareness and appreciation of its presence. This naturally attracts more magic into our everyday lives. While the famous actor and director, Robert Redford, was recovering from a brush with polio as a child, his mother took him to Yosemite. Surrounded by nature's majesty, he experienced a profound sense of connection and hope. It was a turning point for him.

Being in nature can help us to gain clarity in our lives. We tend to lose our sense of purpose in the hectic eddy of activity that characterizes contemporary living. Frequencies generated in natural settings tend to be in balance and harmony. We are positively affected by these good vibrations.

The circle represents a powerful symbol of re-union that we can consciously bring into our homes and offices. We may especially benefit from its powers in healing fractured families. For example, I prescribe for families to sit in a circle face-to-face in the evening and sincerely ask each other, "How was your day?" Simple sharing in circles creates a special magic.[22] The circle has been a centerpiece for Native American ceremonies and rituals.

Healing ourselves with indoor greeneries and outdoor landscaping can create magic. Less stucco, more green is the motto. Researcher Roger Ulrich discovered that post-surgical patients whose rooms faced trees and nature had significantly more rapid rates of recovery. We do not need to be hospitalized to receive such a benefit. We can bring live plants into our kitchens and cubicles to ensure that we have this magic.

Coming Full circle

We come from the earth. When our journey comes full circle, we merge back into the same earth. Earth is magnificent. Earth is magical. Earth is all-embracing. Whenever I visit a sacred place in my sojourns, before I enter into its space, I touch the soil with my hands, bow down and ask permission to explore its power. I also take the soil and rub it on my forehead to energize my third eye, the seat of wisdom. I have gathered, received and shared sacred soils from power centers all over the globe, such as: the Pyramids in Egypt; the Catholic shrine of Santuario de Chimayo in Santa Fe, New Mexico; the Great Wall of China; a Masai village in East Africa; mystical Tibetan caves; the headquarters of Soto Zen in Eiheiji, Japan, Temple of Eternal Peace; Japan's Mt. Hiei and Enryaku-ji Temple within which the inextinguishable Dharma Light has been burning for the past twelve hundred years; and Benares, the oldest city in the world and the city of faith, which is seated along the banks of the Ganges River in India.

While writing this chapter, earth magic was happening — it was serendipity. Susan Saccaro, who was working with me, suddenly said, "Look! There is a full rainbow. One end is coming from the mountains, and the other end is going to the center of the city." It was like a divine bridge. I felt the magic of the earth. What I was writing was manifesting before my eyes.

Once upon a time, Tagore, the Indian poet and Nobel laureate, was writing poetry on his boat by candlelight. Writer's block set in and he was stuck in his mind. Suddenly a gust of wind blew out the candle's flame, and the full moon became his beacon of light. For the first time he experienced the beauty that he was writing about.

The paraclete, the Holy Spirit, always surrounds us and is everywhere. When we touch the sacred soil of the earth and feel the moon's mystery, the romance of earth magic grows and glows.

Reach out, feel and heal.

EXERCISES FOR TRANSFORMATION AND HEALING

1. **Ritual of Respect**: Remember that all places have a soul. Upon entering any abode, we can induce the spirit of the place by offering any gesture of respect. For example, we can light a candle, sprinkle rice or water and welcome the place with gentleness.

2. **A Space for Love**: Whenever we enter our bedrooms, we can say a blessing, such as "I am thankful for this space," regardless of the size and style of our room.

3. **Protecting Home**: Whenever we get into an argument, we should step outside our sacred homes to resolve the conflict. This shields our homes from bringing negative vibrations inside.

4. **Easy Earth Magic**: Use candles, incense and different aromas to uplift our moods and stimulate our senses.

5. **Touching the Earth**: At least once a week, reach out and touch nature. For example, we can soak our hand in soil, rest on a rock, trust a tree or love a leaf.

Notes

1. As a child, I remember participating with my family in the vastukala ceremonies that were conducted by priests inaugurating our new home. This ritual is still practiced by some people living in India today.

2. Refer to *The Garden of Life: An Introduction to the Healing Plants of India*, written by Naveen Patnaik.

3. Additional uses of dowsing will be discussed later in this chapter.

4. The ancient Greek sage, Pliny, coined the term **geomancy** in the first century after the death of Christ.

5. In *Studies in Classical American Literature*, 1923, p. 9.

6. Based on a telephone interview.

7. From Chinese, **feng** meaning wind, and **shui** meaning water.

8. In *The Hidden Effects of Geopathic Disturbances* by D. Brookshire, 1990.

9. Lakhovsky also invented the Multiple Wave Oscillator, a machine used to generate vibrations where individual cells within the organism harmonize with their own frequency and resonate simultaneously to restore balance and health.

10. Refer to Fred Soyka's book, *The Ion Effect: How Air Electricity Rules Your Life and Health*.

11. *Evangeline* by Henry Wadsworth Longfellow.

12. We can call the Environmental Protection Agency for advice on checking for radon levels in our homes.

13. From Dr. Robert Becker's *Cross Currents: The Perils of Electropollution*. A milligauss (mG) is a measurement of the electromagnetic field. Also refer to *The Power of Place: How Our Surroundings Shape Our Thoughts, Emotions, and Actions* by Winifred Gallagher.

14. *American Journal of Industrial Medicine*, 1988.

15. *Raum & Zeit*, Vol. 3, No. 2, 1992.

16. *Electromagnetic Fields: A Consumer's Guide to the Issues and How to Protect Ourselves* by B. Blake Levitt, p. 279.

17. *Warning: The Electricity Around You May Be Hazardous To Your Health: How To Protect Yourself from Electromagnetic Fields*, by Ellen Sugarman.

18. In *Cross Currents: The Perils of Electropollution, The Promise of Electromedicine*, p. 271.

19. Mu metal is the most effective alloy currently being made that shields against magnetic fields. It is quite expensive for the average consumer.

20. Refer to *The Complete Book of Essential Oils and Aromatherapy* by Valerie Ann Worwood .

21. I studied feng shui methods with Master Lin Yun. He is a leading authority on I Ching and feng shui who has a temple in Berkeley, California. Sarah Rossbach, author of *The Chinese Art of Placement*, has done remarkable work to bring this eastern wisdom to the western world in cooperation with Master Yun.

22. Circles have been sacred within all ancient cultures; our modern obsession with rectangular architecture has promoted alienation.

PART THREE

Healing the Spirit

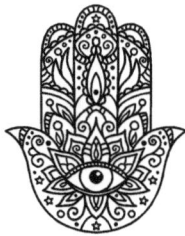

✤

CHAPTER VII

AMUSE-OLOGY

Healing With Laughter

A man needs a little madness,
otherwise he never dares to cut the rope
and be truly free.

—Zorba the Greek

Our last section explored how our bodies can be rejuvenated by sound, food and earth magic — our outer resources. In this section we explore magic within. That is, by changing our outlook, we change the outcome. Our outlook creates our reality.

We are all born with the capacity for amusement. A smile is our first language. In this chapter we explore the relationship between psychophysiology and laughter, "ASAP" applications and what to do to apply the laughter balm.

A GIGGLE IS BORN

The drama of life is a two-act play. The first act is eros, the life instinct, or celebration of life. The second is thanatos, the death instinct, the end of the beginning. My personal penchant for eros is apt to color this chapter in brighter hues rather than darker tones.

I was raised in an ancient Indian culture where life is misery, disease is misery and death is misery. Sermons taught us to renounce all desire, the root of all pain. That created a stoic perspective, and l certainly was stoic. Both culturally and individually, it was as if the champagne of life had gone flat.

After I had an epiphany sitting on that green bench on Brompton Hospital Street in London,[1] my life changed. A shower of hope drenched my soul. The message *to live – give* came to me. The Hebrew word L'chaim, "to life!", literally became my lifeline. I started living rather than trying to survive. We always have choices. It was here that I chose to live and laugh and do everything that enhances **elan**, the joy force.

HOW I LEARNED TO FLY

I then made some changes in my life. For example, I eliminated from my music collection all songs that made a luxury of pain or glorified pathos. I realized that if we pursue sadness, sad things follow. The next thing I altered was my wardrobe. I took out all dark clothing and replaced it with only light and bright fabrics. To me, black symbolized a negation of life, and I wanted to live and laugh.

One rainy afternoon, I was delivering food for a restaurant. When I returned, the owner told me that he could no longer pay me. At that time, I had no other source of income. I then made a series of choices. I thanked him, went home, showered and put on a new shirt. I then went to the theater and saw two comedies to celebrate the loss.

I still watch only happy and uplifting movies. I believe that, in the true romance of life, our *Titanic* does not have to sink, and a plane does not have to crash for an *English Patient* (like me) to have a love affair with life.

I needed to live. And I needed to learn how to fly. I got my wings back by learning to laugh in the face of adversity.

A Peep Into The Past

Once upon a time Jesus was asked, "Who is the greatest in heaven?" Summoning forth a little child from the crowd, Jesus replied, "I tell you the truth, unless you change and become like little children, you will never enter the kingdom of heaven."[2] A child never forgets to laugh.

In the dance of life, when we are humorous we become childlike. Anthropologist Ashley Montagu used the term **neoteny** to describe the journey of growing young. Montagu brilliantly observes that we are suffering from **psychosclerosis**, hardening of the mind. In his masterful book *Growing Young* he shares techniques for recapturing the genius of childhood.

In addressing the Corinthian community, St. Paul retorted, "he should become a 'fool' so that he may become wise."[3] The "fools for Christ"[4] were divinely passionate about their beliefs. Although we know little about them individually, we do know that 42 of these divine fools were canonized in the Russian and Greek orthodox churches. Their passion for Christ's light was so intoxicating that they became known as fools. In this same divine madness, St. Francis was found talking with the birds and the trees and the stars, his personifications of God.

In Sufi[5] tradition, we see the same craziness in celebrating life. The Sufi seekers, when reaching oneness with their divine beloved God, expressed their passion in dervish dances. When watching these ecstatic dances, we can reach the same zenith of passion as the Sufis.

Zen, a form of Buddhism, was the offspring of the marriage between Indian mysticism and Japanese pragmatism. In the tenth century, the Zen master Pu-Tai became the Laughing Buddha. He played with the children and danced like a lunatic. He became the Santa Claus of the Orient. "Give me a penny, give me a penny" was his song. We can place a full-bellied Laughing Buddha statue in our home as an auspicious symbol of wit and wealth .

We can use the Zen searchers as examples in rediscovering our own humor's journey. In becoming masters, they transformed from the cerebral to the celebratory. We, too, can travel toward health as we move from thinking with our heads to expressing with our hearts. It is okay to be a little insane sometimes rather than being a long-faced intellectual. We are all on a mystic path.

If we have a sense of being a nomad like the Sufis, we can transform the demure into dancing.

In Hindu lore, when Chaitanya Mahaprabhu and Mira Bai reached the same level of ecstasy as Godhood, they started dancing and singing with total freedom.

Despite my treks in Tibet, I met the Dalai Lama in my own backyard, in Los Angeles. Even though he was a religious figurehead, to my surprise, he was not serious like other world religious leaders. He exuded neoteny, the childlike quality of exuberance. In his leisure, he became a part-time watch mechanic. From broken watches to broken souls, they came to be fixed by his Holiness. Someone asked the Dalai Lama how he was able to deal with being forced into exile. He compassionately said that he forgave everyone, and that no one can take away his state of mind and joy.

Psychiatrist Viktor Frankl poignantly portrayed his experiences in the Auschwitz concentration camp in his sagacious book, *Man's Search for Meaning: An Introduction to Logotherapy.* Every day he intentionally tried to see something funny and laugh about it, although he could have been annihilated at any moment. Frankl not only used this technique for self-survival, he also infected other prisoners with laughter.

FROM FOOL TO TRICKSTER

The historical fool or clown reemerges in modern society as the trickster. Our protagonist here serves as a social reformer incognito. The trickster is a person who is passionate about something or someone, and is willing to follow it to the nth degree. The Sufi scholar Idries Shah composed a magnificent work entitled *Wisdom of the Idiots*. He explained how the fool becomes the wise man by living the power of dormant wit.

The Trickster is a rebel with a cause. Tricksters promote ingenuity and humor. They want to expose the silliness of the bourgeois, the status quo, the stagnant middle-class world that is based on profit-and-loss morality. The tricksters thrive and move on instinct, and operate on a higher wisdom, the wisdom of happenstance. The modern mystic, George Gurdjieff, was a trickster who used to be called the Sly Master.[6] Gurdjieff helped awaken contemporary man from his somnambulism (sleep walking) by the process of **self-remembering**.

The trickster's approach defies the laws of logic and challenges the status quo. If we could bring this social reformer into the White House and the United Nations, where world peace is serious business, the wisdom of the trickster could trigger a global paradigm shift.

HUMOR AT WORK

Life does not always greet us with clear blue sky. We often find ourselves in a situation with a boss who is a humorless jerk, or a supervisor who is a pain in the neck. What do we do? Let us recall my vignette *How I Learned to Fly* at the beginning of this chapter.

First we find work that we enjoy doing. This is a crucial component of our health. It is no coincidence that the highest rate of heart attack occurs on Monday mornings around 9:00 a.m. because many of .us tend to dread our work. Optimally, we want to be doing the work of our heart's desire. Minimally, we can communicate to clear the bad vibes and, like Viktor Frankl, find something funny to lighten our burdens. It is good, immediate and needle-free medicine.

HEALTH AND HUMOR

A happy heart can create heaven on earth. Do we know that a merry heart literally is good medicine? Researchers are discovering that laughter and longevity have a physiological basis enjoyed both by the "laugher" and the "laughee." Several serious studies highlight the benefits of laughter. Whenever we laugh or feel happy, we release a dose of endorphins, our joy chemicals. Endorphins are similar to morphine, pain relief provided by nature's inner pharmacy.

Lee Berk, DHSc[7] from Loma Linda University, had a funny bone. He conducted a unique experiment. Dr. Berk showed subjects a humorous movie for one hour.[8] Blood samples were then drawn. Results showed decreased levels of chemical stress markers in the blood. Laughing subjects had lower serum levels of epinephrine, dopac, the growth hormone, and cortisol.

Paul McGhee, Ph.D., President of Laughter Remedy,[9] notes that laughter causes increases in immune system functioning marked by elevated levels of different immunoglobulins (IgA, IgG, IgM), complement-3 (immune cells that help pierce through and destroy virally-infected cells), and gamma-interferon, the orchestra leader of the immune system that tells other immune cells when to turn off and on. Although humor and laughter help our immune system to turn on, they are not magic bullets. Even with a healthy dose of humor, traditional treatments should be carefully followed, according to medical advice.

Norman Cousins, author of *Anatomy of An Illness*, likens laughter to internal jogging where different body systems get a workout. Our elevated heart rate stimulates the cardiovascular system. Through raucous laughter, our musculo-skeletal system may become so relaxed that we have a hard time getting out of the chair. Increased rates of inhalation and exhalation provide respiratory benefits.

Allen Klein, a "jollytologist" and author of several books on humor,[10] has a very touching story. His wife, Ellen, had a rare degenerative liver disease, and was hospitalized. Klein and his wife put a male centerfold on the wall in front of her bed. They placed a leaf over his vital part. As days passed, the leaf started shriveling. Ellen later passed away laughing. Since that time, Klein has devoted his life's work to humor, Ellen's legacy.

In writing *The Courage to Laugh: Humor, Hope, and Healing in the Face of Death and Dying*, Klein interviewed 100 individuals during periods of grief. 98% said that humor helped, and that even a little goes a long way. Humor instantly took their minds off their problems, and gave them hope. In a telephone interview with Klein, he explains, "laughter gives us hope, helps us to heal, gives us a different perspective, gives us a reprieve."

ASAP Applications

Klein shows us practical techniques for finding laughter in our lives:

1. Using reminders

2. Teasing ourselves

3. Being around children

Klein personally uses a picture of Woody Allen, his kids, toys, a mask on the wall, oversize greeting cards, and props (e.g., blowing bubbles in traffic) in his humor arsenal. Klein has a note he has posted on his mirror so he sees it daily, "This person is not to be taken seriously."

Making fun of ourselves may not come naturally. For example, Klein is totally bald, and finds humor in calling himself a specialist on balding. He also describes his unique, eulogistic wish, "When I die, I'd like everyone at my funeral to have a jar of bubbles. To me, bubbles represent joy. They have fabulous colors, they're translucent, they're like life, we're here one moment shimmering and shining, then the next moment we're gone."

Observing children, or becoming more childlike, is good medicine. Klein likes to observe children in the airport when his plane is delayed. While most individuals on-hold tend to be stressed, children will sit on the carpet, pull out their toys, and continue with business-as-usual.

Humor not only restores health but can save a life if used in appropriate doses. Norman Cousins had a collagen-degenerative disease. His doctors provided little hope. Refusing to succumb to his somber surroundings, Cousins signed himself out of the hospital and checked into a hotel, where he enjoyed funny movies of the Marx Brothers and Candid Camera episodes. Cousins discovered that "ten minutes of genuine belly laughter had an anesthetic effect and would give me at least two hours of pain-free sleep."[11] Cousins laughed himself back to health.

So what can we learn from this? We can learn to laugh not only in the face of crisis but in day-to-day life. To do things with joy, to do things with simplicity, to do things with fun, to do things with a sense of the miraculous, practice humor in everyday life.

The great Zen master Bankei [12] was asked to prove his ability to perform miracles. Bankei replied, "A fox can do that... but my miracle is when I feel hungry, I eat, when I feel thirsty, I drink."

Humor in Everyday Life

The word **humor** comes from the Latin word **umere**, to flow, to flow effortlessly. When we flow, we come out of our shells . Our culture has taught us that life is serious business, and we develop the dis-ease of being overly-somber. This means that we tend to take the mug shot we see in the mirror too seriously. It was Oscar Wilde who said "life is too serious to be taken seriously."

Humor and laughter liberate us.

What are the ways we can practice humor in everyday life? When life does not treat us well, find the flow, find something funny, smile more, think less, play more, and be a caring trickster.

We all know that every day is not a bed of roses. Some days our car does not start or our spouse does not start. We want to create and life refuses to cooperate. We want to go on a perfect vacation and there is no room at the inn. Does life stop? It can, yet when we cannot change the situation, we can certainly flow with life. We can find something funny in our environment. A grocery store scenario is the perfect place to practice this. When we are standing in line, and the line is going nowhere, we can be in the flow by seeing something funny in the magazine rack beside the cashier. Find the funniest headline. Then talk to a perfect stranger about it. Remember whenever we flow, we are humorous even if we do not laugh.

Do we forecast rain or do we look for the rainbow? Every storm has a surprise. Every sadness has a smile. When our day seems really m-i-s-e-r-a-b-l-e, L-A-U-G-H. There is simplicity in surprises where fun creates freedom. For example, when soap slips out of our hands in the shower, we can pretend we are playing hide-and-seek with Dove. When we are in a hurry and cannot find a shoe, we can remind ourselves of Cinderella and her glass slipper. If we have misplaced our keys we can recall that even the great Masters required some time to discover the keys to the kingdom. Just a slight shift in our outlook can create joy and wonders in ordinary life.

> *Thinking separates us,*
> *smiles unite us.*

A smile is our first form of positive communication. It inherently connects us with others. It is the toll-free bridge to a stranger. When we make our smile our umbrella, it's less apt to rain, and besides, we don't mind getting a little wet now and then. John Diamond, author of *Your Body Doesn't Lie*, discovered that when we smile, or even look at a smile, it strengthens our life energy.

Nietzsche wisely said, "In the true man there is a child concealed, who wants to play." Whenever we do something routine in a slightly different fashion, it allows room for play. When work becomes play, we create fun. If we cannot play with others, whether at home or at work, we can always play with humor by ourselves. For example, in the office, we can sit in our chair from a different direction rather than our habitual direction. We can find an old picture of ourselves as a happy child, and place it in our more-serious workspace. We can hum a happy tune when we enter our home, or whistle while we work.

The purpose of all humor is to laugh with someone not at someone. The trickster is not truly a trickster without compassion. A trickster does not hurt with humor… but heals with humor. That is the essence of the trickster's art. So let us be caring tricksters. For example, we can induce a smile in a grumpy old man, a severe supervisor or a nagging husband using kind words as flowers .

My friend Dr. Paul McGhee[13] is a pioneer, bringing humor into healthcare settings and the workplace. McGhee explains the how-to's of humor. First we decide that we want to have more humor and laughter in our lives. We commit to laugh every day. We then immerse ourselves in humor. For example, McGhee reads his favorite *Farside* comics often, and creates time to spend with funny friends.

When we are having fun, the spirit of play comes out from within. Dr. McGhee prescribes having a good belly laugh at least 5-10 times daily. We can do this when an opportunity for laughter arises, and force ourselves to laugh a little more or a little longer than usual. This may feel uncomfortable at first, but it is a skill we can practice. If something on the outside does not cause our belly to ache, we can laugh on credit.

Did we ever consider selecting language as our next playmate? Puns are fun! I always feel tickled when one of my friends says, "time is fun when you're having flies… if you're a frog." How motivated would we be if someone offered us $1,000.00 each day to identify one or two humorous things? Although it is highly unlikely that such a benefactor exists, the internal rewards we inherit can have greater pay-offs than that.

Dr. McGhee shared a delightful and touching story with me. He and his wife, Amy, met for the first time at a country-western dancing place. They knew they were meant for each other when, on the third dance, their belt buckles got entangled while two-stepping. They literally were joined at the hip, and could not be separated. That was the beginning of the beginning. To this day they remain inseparable.[14]

When Life Gives Us Lemons…

One day in Monte Carlo there was a long line. By chance Charlie Chaplin was there. He discovered there was a Charlie Chaplin look-alike contest in progress. He decided to wait in line as an entrant. When he was called to step forth, the judges awarded him third place. Charlie was awarded third place for being who he was.

Life is full of ironies. One example happened to former president, Ronald Reagan. Mr. Reagan was pursuing his dream to be in a

Hollywood movie. He auditioned for the lead role in the film *The Best Man*. He was rejected because he lacked a presidential persona.

When I was writing as a child, no one took me seriously. Not only that, my teachers scolded me and said, "You can never write." Even my family frequently criticized me when I tried to express myself, chiding, "Can you ever say anything clearly?" One thing I clearly learned then and teach now is when someone says something negative, I do not have to buy into their negativity. If I had bought their message, we would not be reading this book.

The *Guinness Book of World Records* would not exist if everyone believed in limitations. When individuals dare to do what others say cannot be done, they cross the line of the lemon. Lemons happen in every step of life. What can we do when life dishes out disaster and we feel we deserve our dreams, or when we are longing and come up short? These can be turning points. They can be the beginnings of transformation. When we learn to laugh, we begin to turn lemons into liberation.

BUTTERFLY DREAMS

One day the Taoist mystic Chuang Tzu awoke from sleeping. His disciples were amused to see their master dazed and confused. They asked him, "What happened, Chuang Tzu?" To that he replied, "I was sleeping. In a dream, I became a butterfly, but I do not know whether I was a butterfly dreaming I was a man, or a man dreaming that I was a butterfly?" This is the eternal dilemma.

In trying to live, we often miss living. Our modem rush-hour society generates a modem disease, **anhedonia**, a form of apathy where we have lost our ability to feel, to enjoy, to uplift ourselves with pleasure. Many people are suffering from mass anhedonia in modern culture.

When we get what we want, unless we have a sense of gratitude that we tender with thanks-giving, the magic vanishes. It is one thing to have our treasure, and it is another thing to have the capacity to en-joy the treasure. The capacity to en-joy comes from spirit. Spirit is always happy. Spirit is always like a butterfly. Spirit is the smile of life. A truly rich person is that person who can en-joy, not the person who has much but is unable to enjoy.

This very moment stop reading (except for the next sentence!). Let us close our eyes and think of three things we really en-joy. What butterflies do we see?

I was in Thailand. I was staying with the local village people. The younger children were playing outside while the adult children played chess indoors. Farmers had fun in-the-sun plowing the rice paddies. I saw the spirit of **sanuk**, the capacity to have fun, moving throughout all the Thai villages I visited.

When I visit folks in India, people ask me, "Maje me heh?" "Having fun?" This is a popular Indian greeting. Fun is our real wealth. Sometimes back home in southern California I have this "maje me heh" by myself. I spontaneously go to Universal City walk and see tricksters tricking, bubbles blowing, and candy crunching. The children burst out in giggles as the fountain abruptly spurts forth at their feet. Such ambling and rambling cajoles me. Spirit seduces me to join in the divine play. I am reminded of what I have been missing. It reminds me that being saturated in my thoughts and imprisoned in my mind are not my playgrounds of choice.

I come as an adult.
I leave as a child.

LAUGHTER EXPANDS

Life has often given us pain but God has always given us laughter. Even when we feel we have lost everything, we have two constant companions, our smiles and Spirit. Laughter is born when smiles bubble with Spirit.

Life can be bittersweet. We have two choices, to laugh or to cry. In pain when we cry we go inward, with laughter we go outward. When we laugh, the whole world laughs with us, and we can never be alone. Sometimes we can become the holy clown in the divine play of life. In the ministry of life the holy fool is the answer. Darkness and light, sorrow and joy, rejection and love, all are steps in the divine dance. Only the holy fool embraces them all, and plays.

In my search in Tibet, I heard from the inhabitants about a wise idiot, the enlightened teacher, Drukpa Kunley. Kunley awakened people with humor and iconoclastic acts. He practiced the dance of opposites, bringing a sense of sacredness in both the spiritual and the sexual on the road to liberation. *The Divine Madman: The Sublime Life and Songs of Drukpa Kunley*, translated by Keith Dowman, provides intriguing insights about the marriage between the profound and the profane.

RAFOOL'S STORY

Susan and I were quite engrossed in amuse-ology while working on this chapter. At the end of the day, she called a friend. I heard her gasp, as she covered her mouth with her hand. She took me by the shoulders and said, "Rahul, I can't believe what just came out of my mouth! I called you RaFool!!" The next day I shared this with Dr. McGhee during a telephone interview. The good doctor suggested that I take a healthy dose of RaFoolery anytime I felt I was overstocked with lemons, and I started following his prescription. Whenever we become overly serious we laugh by making fun of ourselves. Susan, the good humor lady, reminded me that taking ourselves lightly is good medicine. Norman Cousins once said that, "the great tragedy of life is not death, but what dies inside us while we live."

Life is a celebration when we embrace the moment. Life is mirth when we dance, so let us do the mirth dance and embrace life. Give three hugs and have a big belly laugh .

When Buddha was giving sermons on the mount, he was holding a flower in stillness. Among hundreds of seekers who were gathered around, Mahakasyapa smiled and looked at Buddha. Buddha handed the flower in silence to him. Then he said, "I gave the silent transmission of dharma to smiling Mahakasyapa." Our smile is the gateway to secret blessings if we are willing to receive them.

Laugh with life and
Heal with humor!

RAFOOL'S RULES

1. **God's Taste Buds:** We can celebrate living in the present in
    endless ways, and here's one example. We can intentionally
    slow down when we eat. The next time we have something to
    eat, take five extra minutes to savor the flavor, concentrating on
    the taste and the texture of each morsel. Whenever we are in
    the present, we are with God.

2. **Whistle While We Work**: Literally learn to whistle. Since
    practice makes perfect, we can whistle each time we enter and
    exit our homes. We can whistle in the car, in a restaurant, while
    waiting in lines, or on a long flight while the plane is landing.
    Watch out, it may be contagious!

3. **Disney Delights**: Place a toy or a teddy-bear wherever there is
    serious business. When we feel we are goofing up in life, we can
    have a picture or tangible effigy of Goofy nearby to remind us
    that maybe things are not as serious as they seem. When we
    feel depressed, we can sign our name as Daffy Duck. We can
    make our reservations under the name of Minnie Mouse. (A
    teddy bear is my constant companion in my Saturn automobile
    which I have named Susu.)[15]

4. **It Just Takes A Moment**: When we feel stuck and we are
    miserable, we can close our eyes and tell ourselves that it is our
    last day, and we don't have to worry about a thing. We can take
    a deep breath, open our eyes, and get ready to "rumble" on our
    last day!

5. **Funny Face:** We can go to the nearest mirror, take off our self-
    conscious mask, and find the funny person behind. Pretend we
    are three years old again, and play with our face in the mirror.
    Remember, "the Child is father of the Man."[16]

NOTES

1. See Ch. I *The Healer's Way*, for the story of this epiphany.

2. *Matthew 18: 3.*

3. *1 Corinthians 3:19.*

4. *I Corinthians 4:10.*

5. From the tradition of Islam the Sufis were born.

6. See P.D. Ouspensky's *The Fourth Way* for further details.

7. Refer to The American Journal of Medical Sciences, *Neuroendocrine and Stress Hormone Changes During Mirthful Laughter*, 1989.

8. Gallagher – *Over Your Head*, Paramount Home Video.

9. Based on a telephone interview with Dr. McGhee.

10. Based on a telephone interview with Allen Klein, the author of *The Healing Power of Humor: Techniques for Getting Through Loss, Setbacks, Upsets, Disappointments, Difficulties, Trials, Tribulations, and All That Not-So-Funny Stuff.*

11. *Newsweek*, September 24, p. 98-99, 1979.

12. 1622 -1693.

13. Dr. McGhee is the author of eleven books on humor. Please go to his web-site at www.LaughterRemedy.com to find his latest findings and inspirations, including Humor Your Tumor and Humor in the Workplace.

14. At the time of writing this book, Paul announced that he and his wife are expecting their first child, Skylar.

15. The Brahmaputra, the Ganges, and the Meghna Rivers are all home to a river dolphin called Susu, so named after the in-out breathing sound it makes when surfacing for air. *Dolphins of the World* by Ben Wilson.

16. William Wordsworth's poem *My Heart Leaps Up When I Behold*.

❀

CHAPTER VIII

HEALING THE HEALER

Prana Perspectives and Transformation

The final mystery is oneself.
— *Oscar Wilde*

Pythagorus postulated that completion is represented by the number "3." Energy Medicine takes us through the three inter-dimensional voyages of the healer. The first transit of our journey began with Healing the Mind. The dynamics of healing alchemy occur from within. We saw that we have the power to create an internal pharmacy potent enough to heal anything within the bailiwick of our beliefs. Part Two was the adventure of Healing the Body, rejuvenating our cellular system by food as medicine, sound as vibrational healing, and the biology of environment. The dynamics of Healing the Body are based on our harmony with external resources. The culmination of the Healer's Journey is Part Three, Healing the Spirit, a return to within. The soul heals itself by amuse-ology, the laughter prescription, as we have seen in the previous chapter.

PRANA PERSPECTIVE

Healing the Healer is the palette of this chapter where, by changing our perspective, we infuse prana (the breath of life) and empower ourselves. We can eat a balanced diet, and create the perfect environment, but if our outlook is not imbued with prana perspective we cannot heal.

We are born with a mind mired in a collective perspective. The collective perspective is derived from our need for safety, security and stability. For our inner healer to emerge, we need to shift from a collective to a prana perspective. Prana perspective is based on personal longing, meaning, and quest. Our soul wants to play. Our soul wants to find a soulmate to play with. Our soul wants to have deep fulfillment in our ordinary experiences.

The process of transformation begins when we reunite our prana perspective with our soul. Transformation must happen in order to give ourselves a new birth. In India, a brahman is a person who has undergone this journey. Brahman means "twice-born." However, in contemporary Indian society, the twice-born brahmanas have lost their symbolic meaning. It has become a form of caste dogma based on family of origin.

Our first birth is our physical birth. A shift in consciousness enables the birth of the soul-self. The realization of our soul-self is a profound awareness happening today, among men and women in their healers' journeys.

We change our world when
We change our perspective.

Soul Searching

We are all healers, we are wounded healers — wounded by chaos, wounded by separation, wounded by dis-ease, wounded by fractured families, wounded by loneliness. All these injuries come from the same source, starvation of soul. Psychologist Carl Jung described the wounded healer as the wounded physician based on Greek mythology. "It is his own hurt that gives the measure of his power to heal."[1]

When we need to heal something, we must give willingly the very thing we desire for ourselves. For example, when we want a new life, and we want love in our life, we must go and give completely by sharing and by inspiring someone. That is where healing happens.

A healer has to pass through the full circle. Where there is pain, there is chaos. Where there is pain, there is heaviness. These are our reminders to change. "Oard ka haad se gujarjana he dawa ho jana hea."[2] Pain itself becomes a medicine when it passes through a threshold. Our pain threshold varies from person to person. It also depends on which threshold we choose to cross.

How do we change? Robert Frost described this process, "the only way out is through." As healers, we must give the very thing we desire:

Give what we do not have.
Give what we want.

When we live in a ring of negativity, we are not a healer. One day I had an argument that spiraled into upheaval. There seemed no way out to break the ring of negativity. I could not sleep with that upset. At that point, my greatest moment of vulnerability, my soul swirled into awareness. I surmounted and broke the ring of negativity by reaching out to give a hug. Healing instantly began to flow.

THE ENERGY OF EMOTIONS

Dis-ease is a reminder of our loss of power. Loss of power breeds helplessness. Helplessness depresses the immune system and drains our life force. We are in constant relationships. If not with others, with ourselves. The loss of power in relationships manifests as dis-ease. In my experience in Energy Medicine, betrayal manifests as chronic back pain. Lung congestion, chronic colds and allergies represent the repression of creativity. Abdominal distress is literally a distrust of others. Headaches, neck and shoulder pain are unresolved responsibilities.

Obstacles in the flow of money block the flow of sexual energies. I frequently see and hear these patterns of distress in others.

We will begin to explore how to heal the emotional center of these particular symptoms. For example, people who have back problems need to let go of critical and betraying people in their lives, and to create a new circle of supportive friends. Unless and until this emotional energy is released and rejuvenated, our long-term healing will not happen. Mere physical interventions, such as herbs, body manipulation and taking medication are not enough.

A MIRACLE OF HEALING

Laura Evans from Florida came to see me in California before Thanksgiving, 1998. She was first diagnosed with breast cancer in the fall of 1988. At the time of her initial diagnosis, Laura had lost her marriage. In her words:

You see in the Fall of 1988, I was diagnosed with breast cancer, at that time I also went through a divorce. It was a very challenging time of my life. I did recover and went on living my life without any significant change in my lifestyle. In the Fall of 1996, I found out I have a recurrence. At that time, I was determined to change my lifestyle. Last Spring during a seminar called THE DAY OF THE AWAKENING at the Miami Arena, Rahul Patel, the Energy Healer, rendered healing services. While doing healing services, he announced his phone number. I was constantly seeking and getting Rahul's healing techniques on the phone until finally I met with Rahul on November, 1998 in Los Angeles, California. There, with my consent, he laid his hands on my chest area and my whole body during a healing session. It was a great experience, since then I feel great. I have more energy. I have changed my diet and include daily prayer, fasting and meditation, as he suggested, including my other medical practice (doctor's advice). I have also experienced growth in every area of my life. Rahul, through it all, I have found that very special person "LAURA" again.

I thank you Rahul from my heart for all the healing sessions and your divine therapeutic touch that you offered, saved my life. Sincerely, Laura Evans[3]

MAP OF HEALING

There is a direct corollary between loss and disease. The first thing I always notice before a breakdown is a loss of personal power. In the fall of 1988 Laura went through a divorce at the same time she was given a diagnosis of breast cancer.

The second thing I observe is that after a breakdown, if healing happens, stars emerge in our lives. The first nova[4] is a **radical shift** in our approach to life. Next comes a constellation, a series of **epiphanies.** The breakdown of personal power makes us dis-ease-prone. The person who heals is the person who goes through an instantaneous shift.[5] For example, instantly letting go of a person whom we have allowed to steal our power. The second shift is epiphanies, instant insights. It happens anywhere, while sleeping, driving the car, taking a shower or talking on the phone. We do not have to be on the road to Damascus to experience an epiphany.

Our angels speak to us as a reminder, "Pay attention." Attend to the epiphany and change. When we listen to the message contained in this opening, we typically experience a 180 degree shift in our perspective. When we "see the light," things never look the same again.

I clearly saw in Laura that she could heal because she had the life instinct. Her willingness to do anything was her turning point. In 1998, Laura made radical changes in her lifestyle and relationships. She also started listening to her soul. I suggest that she practice daily prayer and meditation to deepen this burgeoning relationship with her soul. Laura was ready to receive. At that point, I invited her to spend a day of healing with me.

Healing usually happens when we have a determination to receive it. The sun was setting in the late autumn Los Angeles sky. I laid my hands on Laura. With deep compassion, I shared the healing energies of therapeutic touch, the gift that God had given me. I saw a plane taking off in the silhouette of the orange sun as the healing was taking place. I had a sudden epiphany. The plane was now soaring against the full sun, as I shared with Laura, "You are free to relive your life. You are on a healing path."

January 19, 1999 Laura had a follow-up mammogram. According to her doctor, "The right side is normal. The left side appears normal without any undue lumpiness or other changes that would suggest recurrence. In the area of her sensory symptoms, I can palpate nothing abnormal."

EMPOWERING THE HEALER

Laura experienced a radical shift when she "…found that very special person 'LAURA' again." Rediscovering our authentic self is the beginning of our healer's journey. Laura also translated her epiphany into action. That is, she began giving the very thing she desired. In Laura's words, "healing is helping others heal themselves. Today, I am very active in the community helping others go through the challenges they face when they are first diagnosed with breast cancer."

With what other ways can we empower our healer within? UCLA researcher Shelley Taylor, Ph.D., authored the fascinating book *Positive Illusions: Creative Self-Deception and The Healthy Mind*. Dr. Taylor concluded that healthy people seem not to see things as they are but see things as they would like them to be. One of the keys to health is the positive perception of reality that enhances self-esteem and gives a sense of control.

As healthy people, we can create an exaggerated confidence in ourselves, and harbor endless optimism in our potential. I interpret this as positive illusion. By seeing things not as they are but as we desire them to be, we can make our dreams come true. Einstein experienced this as creative imagination. Einstein said, "The gift of fantasy has meant more to me than my talent for absorbing knowledge." For Einstein, fantasy was the positive illusion that enabled him to break through the limitations of the status quo, and to free himself from the prison of the mind.

When people are given exactly the same diagnosis of a life-threatening disease, they may react differently. The outcome is based on their perception. The ones who believe they will live, live. It naturally follows that in order to change the result, we must first change our perception.

Our imaginations become crushed at such an early age. We are taught that using our imagination is fanciful and unproductive. We need to resurrect one of our greatest assets in healing, our imagination, to create the perfect mental picture of our utopia, a vivid image of our perfect partner, perfect lifestyle, perfect home and perfect adventure. We can live as if we have it all.

Psychic induction is the quickest way to break the ring of negativity and empower ourselves and others. Psychic induction is a process of giving and receiving empowerment.

As we have seen, the loss of power is the beginning of dis-ease. To reverse the dis-ease process, we can initiate an instant communication with sincere kindness. For example, we can begin by asking, "How is the weather?," or, "how is your day?" If no one is around, we can even chat with a stranger or a telephone operator. This is the best way to start psychic induction. Talking about day-to day matters, like greetings and the weather, builds a natural bridge. This connection brings a surge of power that causes a shift. By practicing psychic induction when we feel powerless, when we feel hurt, when we feel stalled, we release the flow of power.

FIND THE FLOW

Healing happens when we enjoy what we are doing so much that we lose a sense of time. Find something that creates the flow, such as playing a favorite sport, being with a loved one, creating something new, reading a book we cannot put down, getting lost in music, or simply flowing with our beingness—doing nothing—it all creates a sense of enthusiasm. The word enthusiasm comes from the Greek words en-theos, in God, to flow with the energy of God within.

We enhance our health by creating flow. The famous psychologist Abraham Maslow called this **peak experience**. Maslow has been a lone ranger in the field, being the first to incorporate the psychology of health versus pathology. Prior to Maslow, psychologists analyzed dis-eases of the mind, and tend to continue this emphasis in contemporary practice. The healthier we are, the more peak experiences we have. Peak experiences are thrills we can weave into our daily lives. And I am not talking about cheap thrills! In *Healthy Pleasures*, Robert Ornstein, Ph. D. and David Sobel, M.D., integrate illustrations of this in a brilliant fashion .

Researcher Avram Goldstein of Stanford University developed a scale to measure thrills, the sense of excitement. In a survey, respondents rated a number of thrills, including: physical exercise (36%),[6] unexpected events (63%), sex (70%), beauty in art and nature (87%), scenes in literature, theater and movies (92%) and music (96%).

There are countless ways in which we can create flow. Silence for two in love may be equivalent to a roller-coaster ride for one. For many, being close to G-O-D or a D-O-G is basking in an ongoing, loving relationship that triggers peak experiences and creates a flow. When we find the flow, we find the joy that nurtures our soul.

From Persona to Person

All our lives we are entrapped by our personalities. The word personality comes from the word *persona* and the Etruscan root meaning, "mask." Society creates masks for maintaining order. In the journey of the healer, we do not need any mask between ourselves and God. In fact, our mask is the barrier. By living our essence we return to the person who we truly are. Our essence is what we are born with — our capacity to love, our longing for oneness and our ability to find meaning in our lives. By listening to the voice of our heart, we embrace our eternal essence.

> *Persona is a creation of the public.*
> *Person is a creation of God.*

Seeking the Song of Life

We are all born with something special. There is no other person like us today in this world. We are the signature of God. There is a song that we are born with.[7] Every organization, and society at large, may appear to be against the personal melody of our individual lives. We can find that by transcending any members of our family who may be suppressing us, and by releasing disharmonious persons from our life we can come to the voice of our heart. When we live our voice, no matter what others think of us, we feed power to our souls. We can follow our special talent, our joy, the very thing that makes us happy.

In my journey, I was born into a business family. There was business before me, and there was business after me. I was the family drop-out. In seeking my song of life, I explored the world, and found that the whole world was my family. In following my song, I came close to God, and received the empowerment that has allowed me to utilize my gifts of healing.

A healer is within all of us, if we are only willing to listen to the special melody of our life and sing it. "Singing" means to actualize our special talent and celebrate it as the essence of our life. One of the ways God speaks to us is by giving us a song.

When we sing our song,
we come close to God.

How to Heal Ourselves and Others

In the previous seven chapters, we have seen how to: change our mind, breathe for energy healing, create healing sounds, choose foods as good medicine, change the environment to create healing energies, laugh to liberate our souls and transform by altering our prana perspective.

We heal ourselves when we find ourselves. We love ourselves when we fully embrace ourselves. We can only love others when we love ourselves first. The healer in each of us can activate healings in others, but we need to begin by loving ourselves. Here are practical ways to get started. Take a moment and sit in silence, lie down and surrender. Look in the eyes of a child or touch a pet. We can choose to change the vibrations from stagnation to serenity, and concentrate on something loveable about ourselves. These simple techniques can provide a turning point.

Even in our darkest hour, when we feel truly awful about ourselves, there is something loveable in all of us. We must find that glint, whether or not we feel like it. Whatever the crisis, no matter its breadth and depth, bringing the flame of love back to our own hearts can rekindle our prana perspectives.

See a new vision at that point of love. Paint a picture of health, harmony and happiness. Silently assign ourselves a small love job. For example, "This is what I'm going to do today in my love job. Pay a pending bill, clean up a drawer, clean out an old closet, rearrange my shoes or write a memo to myself." The flow of love for ourselves and others stops when we are caught in an impasse — an impasse of money, an impasse of blame, an impasse in relationships. Once we overcome the trauma of impasse by determination and love, only then can the life force flow anew.

> *A little effort goes a long way*
> *in the healer's way.*

It is like a thin silk thread of hope. Once we catch a glimpse of clarity in our crisis we need to act upon that clarity immediately, with no postponement. This is how we create new pathways for healing. The small voice within and outer coincidences will lead us to our next step, when we are willing to listen and follow.

The things we have acquired are merely possessions until we begin to share. When we share what we have with compassion it becomes eternal wealth. When our sharing is heartfelt, our wealth can never be taken away. The angel of healing, Raphael, is looking over us.[8]

> *Compassion, not knowledge, transforms.*

In Buddhist tradition, a bodhisattva is a seeker on the path of enlightenment who experiences permanent bliss. The bodhisattva comes back to share with compassion. Compassion and love heals the bridge between two minds, between two bodies, between two hearts, between two souls. Knowledge does not change completely if there is no compassion. When a book touches something inside us, or a speaker or a stranger or an animal looks in our eyes with compassion we transform with love.

A BUTTERFLY KISS

There is a moving story of healing by compassion in the animal kingdom. It touches me every time I talk about it. Joseph Krutch refers to a letter in *The Countryman*, a popular British quarterly. The tale tells of a person who saw a parasite hanging on the eye of a butterfly. The person tenderly removed the parasite. The butterfly touched the person's hand with its mouth. I believe the butterfly offered this kiss as a token of gratitude.[9] It is possible that nature can demonstrate this compassion in trees and birds, even in rocks, if one has the eye of the beholder. Jesus said, "lift the stone and you will find me, cleave the wood and I am there."

THE HEALING TOUCH

Touch is the first and the essential language of healing. Our first communication of love comes with a touch. It can even conquer our greatest fear, assuaging feelings of abandonment. When we integrate touch with compassion, we gain access to an eternal reservoir of health called the healing touch of **energy transference** (ET). ET enables deep-rooted, painful memories to release and the recipient often experiences a positive, internal shift. Although there are many ways of doing it, the only qualification we need for practicing ET is compassion.

We begin by closing our eyes, folding our hands and listening to our inner voice. As healers, we serve as conduits, empty vessels for Spirit. Clarity of intention and strength of will allow us to become instruments of health. The next step is to rub our hands together until we feel a tingling sensation of warmth. We then place our hands on the part of the body that needs healing. Our inner voice will show us where to start and how to proceed. Energy always flows from left to right, so begin with the left side (feminine, receptive energies) and proceed to the right side (masculine, giving energies).

Observe the breathing patterns of the healer and healee to ensure they are synchronized. I call this **entering the pulse**. This is the power exchange between the healer and the healee that enables the healer to become a channel for spirit. The emptier we are as a healer, the more beneficial it is for the healee. The empathy of touch teaches us when to move on to other parts, if we do not dwell on details of the mind but flow with the compassion of our heart. Once we complete all the areas of the body, we must be grateful for having the opportunity to heal because healing is divine.

ET is a sacred art that has been practiced throughout the history of humankind. ET can work on human beings only if they desire and believe. But ET always works on pets and plants because they do not have logic, they have magic. It is our thinking caps that are the obstacles between ET and healing. That is why ET works with some people, and not with others.

We can enhance ET by working in alignment with natural energies. When we are healing male clients, we can face our sessions to the north. When we are healing female clients, we can face south. South brings the warmth of fire and north brings the dampness of cold. We need to assess the male-female balance within the individual's energy field. For example, a person's challenge may be masculine although she is in a female body. In that case, we face south. When we are in the process of shedding the past, we face west. When we want to create a new surge of energy, face east.

After completing ET, we start from the stomach and move our hands clockwise to help release suppressed emotions . Next by placing our hand in the area between the stomach and the chest just below the sternum, we can reactivate the will. We can then release creativity by bringing both hands gently to the chest area, after asking the consent of the healee.

We can give direct ET by having the healee put the tip of their tongue on the upper arch of the roof of their closed mouth. The healer rhythmically taps their middle finger on the healee's thymus. According to John Diamond, author of *Your Body Doesn't Lie* tapping the thymus energizes us.[10]

ET is completed by putting both hands over the eyes and the forehead, touching the crown of the head with our fingertips. When we touch a child with love it is ET. It is our intention and compassion which makes it work.

Conducting healing in the silence of home or the serenity of nature can be effective based on personal preferences. Many times tears will flow, or we need to go to the bathroom more frequently, both are signs of releasing old toxins. The effect of ET may last a day, a night, a week, or a lifetime, depending upon the synergy of intention and compassion.

NEW PRANA PERSPECTIVES

Prana perspective is a transcendence of consciousness that dissolves past conditioning. We typically function in a mechanical manner that is constricting. Our brain has set neuropathways that tend to keep us in old habits. The first step in changing our destiny is to become aware of our mechanical habits. Then we can make new, conscious choices. These choices incite new electrochemical signals and we build new pathways of prana perspective. Then our old paradigms and behavior patterns begin to transform.

Let's play the Newton game. When we are looking at an apple and a scientist takes a PET (positron-emission tomography) scan of our head, a certain part of our brain lights up. When the apple is put aside, we close our eyes and imagine the apple, the same area of our brain will light up. In the hologram of our brain, it does not matter whether an object is physically present. We create the image in our mind. Visualization activates the totality of our neurocircuitry which in turn affects our emotional and physical bodies.

Perception creates possibility.

When our brain is exposed to the same humdrum, the same routine, the same nagging voices every day, it goes through sensory anesthesia. In day to day life, we are anesthetized to spiritual matters and our own essence. We are numb to joy and bliss and ecstasy, the very things we desire. We suffer from mass anhedonia.

EINSTEIN'S HEAD

Marian Diamond, Ph.D.[11] and a team of researchers discovered what made Einstein unique. They literally opened his mind and found more glial cells per neuron than the average head. Glial is Greek for "glue." These cells nurture and protect neurons, the electrochemical couriers of communication. Dr. Diamond discovered that being in an environment full of novel stimuli virtually bolsters our brain. In my understanding, exposure to such an enriched environment can create new neuropathways that can heal us if we allow ourselves to see newness. By seeing new things in everyday life, even in ordinary circumstances, we practice our new prana perspectives.

Oliver Cromwell and Lord Byron had something in common. Their brain weight was 2200 grams. Einstein's brain weighed only 1400 grams.[12] It is not size that matters. But in gray matter, it does matter how we use it.

THE ALCHEMY OF ALCATRAZ

Alcatraz is a prison located on an island in the middle of San Francisco Bay. It had the reputation of being the toughest prison from which to escape. A man was given a lifetime sentence. In his cell, one day a bird fell down in front of him. He nurtured the bird back to health, learning everything he could about birds in the process. By the genius of his creativity, he was immortalized as the Birdman of Alcatraz. He "escaped" prison by activating his imagination. Everyone brought birds to him for treatment. He became a leading authority on ornithology. He transformed hades into heaven by creating an enriched environment in his mind.

We can convert our everyday existence into a kaleidoscope of creativity. We need to change our perspective and intentionally see something new in everyday life. We can see mud outside the window, or admire the reflection of the moon in the mud. By creating thrills and living in an inner, enriched environment, we can reframe our prana perspective.

THE HEART OF TRANSFORMATION

The gift we are all freely given is the ability to transform. When we transform ourselves and others we fulfill God's prophesy. How do we transform?

Once upon a time a sparrow collapsed from the sky, and fell into a cage at a Swiss zoo. The resident chimpanzee found the tiny bird, put it gently in her hand, and cradled the crashed flier. To the zookeeper's amazement, the chimpanzee then passed the sparrow to him.[13]

We transform when we matter to someone, or someone matters to us. We do not have to be physically close to a person. Just having the perception that someone out there cares for us motivates us to change. Whatever happens to us can affect another person deeply, and creates the synergy of transformation. This love, this sense of belongingness is the essence of change.

This love is not for sale. We can buy pure water, pure air and organic carrots. But we cannot purchase an organic sense of belonging.

Reach out and touch someone.
Reciprocity heals.

EXERCISES FOR TRANSFORMATION AND HEALING

1. **Appreciating Beauty**: For one week, find at least three things every day that instill a sense of beauty. Post these beauty tips on the refrigerator. A beauty a day keeps the doctor away. Seeing beauty is a great anti-aging prescription.

2. **Open Outlook**: Take our watch off and put it in a drawer. Put away our paper and pens. Turn down the ringer on the telephone. Now we are ready for our sensorium experience. Taste the toast. Sip the melting sorbet. Touch texture. Be present with full senses without getting caught up in narrow details. We can open our outlook and play sensorium with oneself or others.

3. **Inspire and Share**: Find something uplifting or moving that touches our hearts. Then share this with another person. Even our pets and plants will be happy recipients of our sharing. We also can allow ourselves to receive inspiration from others.

4. **Miracle Bag**: Write the most powerful thing that we desire on a small slip of paper. Fold it with reverence, and place it in a special bag or box. As we add other symbols of power to this bag or box, we are making direct deposits to our destiny. It will en-rich all of our days.

5. **Power Touch**: Reach out and touch a near or dear one. We can even touch the picture of a loved one to energize ourselves. Touch whatever brings personal power (precaution: parental discretion advised). Send ET, whether near or far, and they will receive it.

Notes

1. Refer to *The Practice of Psychotherapy: Essays on Psychology of the Transference and Other Subjects*, 1966, translated by R.F.C. Hull and edited by William McGuire, p. 116.

2. Urdu language of the Middle East.

3. Dated February 9, 1999. Used in text with full permission from the writer, Laura Evans.

4. A nova is a newly-exploded star that suddenly becomes visible in the night sky.

5. Change is gradual. Transformation is instantaneous. Instant transformation is the only transformation. However, it may require a lot of effort to prepare the soil for transformation.

6. See *Physiological Psychology*, 1980.

7. Lawrence LeShan, Ph.D. repeatedly used this technique in his therapy with cancer patients. Please refer to his book *Cancer as a Turning Point: A Handbook for People with Cancer, Their Families, and Health Professionals*.

8. I am inspired to recommend having a full-ceiling mural of Raphael in our home for around-the-clock companionship.

9. A sensitive reference can be found in *When Elephants Weep: The Emotional Lives of Animals* by Jeffrey Masson, Ph.D. and Susan McCarthy.

10. The thymus gland can be found by locating a slight protrusion of the breast bone 1-2 inches below the top of the sternum.

11. Department of Physiology-Anatomy, University of California, Berkeley.

12. Found in *Brainfood: A Provocative Exploration of the Connection Between What You Eat and How You Think* by Jean Marie Bourre, M.D.

13. Refer to *When Elephants Weep: The Emotional Lives of Animals*, Jeffrey Masson, Ph.D., and Susan McCarthy.

❊

CHAPTER IX

THE SPIRIT OF POSSIBILITIES

Holographic Healing

The soul is a fiery eye...
from the eternal centre of nature.
— *Jacob Bohme*

Spirit can be felt, not proven. The most beautiful things in life can only be experienced. Spirit is the diamond in the sky, and our cherished wishes can make it glow. We are the akashic record,[1] the celestial collection of our entire possibilities. We long for glory, although we often remain unaware of our own power to bring magic. We want some god or goddess outside ourselves to come and *poof*, create the magic for us. However, we are magicians. We create the bridge across possibilities. We often have been disheartened and broken in our dreams. This helplessness can be the seed of new beginnings.

When I died and saw the light, the Voice distinctly gave me two alternatives in my hologram of possibilities. One was to close the chapter of life and give up my body, the other option was to return and walk the path of will — to do anything and everything to enhance prana. This required me to surrender to Spirit.

Life is a gift from Spirit. What we do with our life is our gift to Spirit. We are given a life, a chance to love, to find meaning and a chance to share our deepest aspirations. The look of love in someone's eyes, the smile of an angel, a tender touch and en-joy-ment all are notes in the symphony of our soul that resonates because of spirit.

In this chapter we explore the map of manifesting our possibilities through the synergy of *will* and *surrender*. We will outline the practice of daily rites of the Spirit and how we filter the hologram of healing by transcending the dance of opposites. We determine our destiny by how we are living today. By finding ways of harnessing our hidden potential we create the hologram of healing.

WILL AND SURRENDER TO SPIRIT

We are often fragmented in our actions but we are whole in our vision. We have multiple broken selves. Our many "I's" weaken our will. For example, one part of us loves, and one part of us hates. We decide to make a fresh start yet obstacles dampen our courage.

Our warrior aspect is our will. To strengthen our warrior, we must be aware of our inner voice. We must act upon its guidance immediately or the cacophony of fragmented voices will soon begin to drown out the still small voice within.

Will is our act of conviction. It is a journey of becoming masters in creating our own destiny. Let us take two examples. We are all singers, yet we tend to sing in hidden ways, in the shower, in the car, or in our heads. How many times have we wanted to be a writer or a poet, only to end up with a heap of crumpled paper in the trash can at our feet? Why do we so often feel that we have become a caravan of broken dreams?

How do we transform this caravan into a parade of joyous possibilities? By acting in the present moment with our vision we can imbibe will. For example, by acting instantly on our vision, even when it is not fully-formed, we trigger the flow of power in our lives.

Here is how we begin the power-will practice. Go to the bedroom and determine what needs to be done. Do we see a need to clean, rearrange, or replace? It may not be the bedroom we need to redo. We can take an inventory of our relationships, and do a little spring cleaning. Instead of postponing, the key is to act upon it. For example, we can call someone new we met with whom we felt some type of affinity. Settling unpaid bills or debts enables a fresh flow of financial resources to enter into our lives. A simple act of will changes our vibrations and opens us to new possibilities. The secret is finding clarity within our vision and using our will to take action.

Vision generates clarity.
Action generates will.

There is a process that will come to us when we are ready to act upon it. Messages from Spirit come in many different forms.[2] When we are open, we do not have to force things to happen. Things will happen at just the right time, as long as we remain open.

Meir Schneider was declared legally blind at the age of seven, but he refused to surrender to blindness. He had a burning will to see. I believe that his intense will forged new optical pathways. His extensive and unique exploration of sight gave him his vision back. He went on to earn a driver's license and a Ph.D. Dr. Schneider now teaches his methodology of vision and healing world wide. The will is the way, even when we are told that we cannot see.

We have various centers that we can mobilize to access our energies: an emotional center, a physical center, an intellectual center, and an intuitive center. We often experience conflict and imbalance within these energy centers. For example, when we are moving furniture, we are in our physical center. The moment we experience emotional distraction, we begin to divert our physical energies to the emotional center. This can rob us of our physical energy and create fragmentation of different "I's." By the process of self-remembrance, we can integrate the fragmented "I's," and gain full access to our will power.[3]

Suzanne Kobasa, Ph.D.[4] and a team of researchers conducted a study of AT&T executives who were going through organizational restructuring. They identified "hardy" subjects as those who exhibited three primary characteristics: commitment, control, and challenge.

Under significant stress, hardy individuals sustained a positive relationship with their roles (commitment). They maintained their personal power, and looked for ways they could improve the situation (control). They also responded to change with flexibility and became invigorated rather than defeated (challenge).

How do we create will? We go against the drift, listen only to our inner convictions, and act upon them. This is how we activate the power of will. By seeing challenges as inspiration and growth, and by exercising our conviction as commitment to growth, we can regenerate our lost and fragmented will.

SPIRIT IN ACTION

Will is nothing without spirit. Spirit is our healer aspect. Spirit is the divine fuel for everything we do. It is the super-glue that holds us together eternally.

Spirit is our genetic inheritance. That inheritance cannot be destroyed. Spirit surmounts all challenges, and contains our **hologram**, our blueprint of possibilities. We are all born with the divine hologram, each one of us having unique talents. Our hologram is the pathway we instinctively know yet have difficulties following. Our inner intention, called yi, in Chinese, is the way to empower our spirit.

A star shines when we see love in someone's eyes for the first time. "There was a star danced, and under that was I born."[5] Spirit is that star. Spirit leads us on the journey to find our soulmates.[6] We have many soulmates. Whenever we find a "special" exchange of meaning with someone or something that becomes a driving force, we have found a soulmate. All kinds of love are the best kinds of love. We tend to see lack when actually there is more than enough to go around. There is a plethora of possibilities awaiting us.

Spirit will guide us if we are willing to take the risk of letting go of our defenses and doubts. We must be willing to let go of all of our don'ts: don't talk to strangers, don't trust, don't dream. We can be the god or goddess of possibilities at our own risk. (precaution: parental discretion not advised).

A god or goddess is a soulmate who is willing to play, an eternal enchanter who flows freely with life. It is this quality that allures us, the synergy of Spirit and mystique. When we first join the god and goddess within ourselves, we then are prepared to unite with another soulmate.

Spirit provides us with the power to achieve super human feats, such as out-of-body (OOB) experiences, dream-talk, premonition, deja vu, near-death experience (NDE), clairvoyance, psychic surgery, fire-walking and energy transference (ET). In everyday life, we all exhibit a glimmer of the same supernatural power. For example, the next time we go to our mailbox, if we close our eyes and imagine who has written us a letter, we will be surprised how often our hunches are correct. We can practice this when we are waiting for an elevator by visualizing which elevator is going to open first. Wait and see how close our imagery comes to reality.

During my Tibetan sojourn, I heard about **gtummo**, a mystical practice of creating heat by harnessing the tremendous power of spirit. Monks sit naked in freezing temperatures with wet sheets wrapped around them. By altering their consciousness and accessing power through meditation, they are able to dry wet sheets in approximately 30 minutes.[7] Spirit is so powerful that all things are possible.

God said to the people of Israel, "Fear not, for I have redeemed you... when you walk through the fire, you will not be burned" (Isaiah 43:1,2). I literally tested this belief. I walked barefoot on fire several times without training in Santa Fe, New Mexico in 1995. I know that Spirit is always there. Whether sitting in cold, walking on fire, or standing in the tepidity of today, Spirit is here, there and everywhere, with each and with every one of us.

RITES OF SPIRIT

If we are born with omnipresent Spirit, how can we access this in daily life without going to Tibet or Santa Fe? Spirit is our very nature. We never depart from Spirit, nor does Spirit ever depart from us. Our awareness is the missing link that can cause us to feel disconnected. I propose simple rites to reawaken our awareness of Spirit in daily life: owning our selves, listening to our inner voice, acting more on essence, letting go of critical people, seeing and celebrating the sacred, being aware of synchronicity and practicing duaah.

First we own ourselves. We reclaim our desires and dreams, our youthfulness and our yearnings. We have been rejected, dejected and ejected repeatedly in our life's dramas. We can break this pattern and create ourselves anew.

Gerald Coffee was a Naval officer who was shot down and held prisoner for seven years during the Vietnam War. His cell, one of the notorious *tiger cages*, was neither tall enough for him to stand, nor long enough for him to lie down and stretch out. The Viet Cong attempted to break his spirit. Coffee did not yield to his oppressor's intention. He reclaimed himself by communicating with his fellow prisoners using Morse Code and tapping on the walls. He triumphed through Spirit by reciting inspirational pieces from Rudyard Kipling. He also began to teach himself a foreign language using Morse code. Coffee's method is beautifully illustrated in *Beyond Survival*. His solace came from his conversations with God. In his darkest hours, he prayed, "God, help me use this time to get better." This simple line helped bring him back to himself and gave him enough strength to live for tomorrow.

We are inmates in the prison of our limited awareness. We are constantly struggling to free ourselves from that bondage. Rousseau once said, "Man is born free but is everywhere in chains." How do we break the chains that bind us? By listening to our inner voice, especially when we wake up and when we go to sleep. At these times, we tend to be in a twilight zone, where our mind quiets down and the voice of our heart can be more easily heard. We can keep writing materials next to our bed and record the messages that come to us.

Someone once asked Bach how he composed music. He replied that when he awakened, it was there. The question was not how to compose but how not to crush it when he got up. Like Bach, our visions are whole. Yet how many times throughout our day do we crush them?

Another way to own our selves is to act on essence and not on personality. As we discussed, personality is our mask and person is our essence. In order to find our essence, we can recall the things that we dreamed of and enjoyed doing when we were young. We can also reclaim our selves by doing things that give us a feeling of freedom. As a child, I used to love drawing and being with nature. I loved listening to the birds, trees and silence. Now, doing healing brings me to the same serenity that I found in nature as a child. As a child I lived the dream of a man.

Another effective way of finding our authentic selves is letting go of critical people around us. Nothing is changed for the better by being critical. To the contrary, it is destructive. Beware of well-wishers who are critical (e.g., "I'm only doing this for your own good"). Following our hearts brings us closer to our real selves. It is perfectly all right to make "mistakes." At least they are our own. Often times what we perceive as mistakes are stepping stones to transformation.

Once we find our authentic selves by these processes, we will be ready to change many mechanical things, from our wardrobe to our vocabulary. Often times we find ourselves attached to possessions or perceptions that no longer serve us. The key is to let go of the past. For example, we can give away old "stuff" as we are reclaiming our essence. This emptying allows a new energy of joy to flow in.

Another rite of Spirit is seeing and celebrating the sacred. "The way you make love is the way God will be with you."[8] We can find something sacred in everything. It all depends on our spiritual eyesight. The ordinary and the average can become extraordinary when we uncover our creativity.

In Zen, in the first stage of the journey, mountains are mountains, and rivers are rivers. When we are struggling to find our authentic selves, the mountains are not mountains, and the rivers are not rivers. When we liberate ourselves by finding our authentic selves, the mountain again becomes the mountain, and the river again becomes the river. But the first and the last mountains are different because we have gone through the journey of discovering our soul en route. Now we can see the sacred in the mundane. A pebble on the sand, an acorn beneath the oak tree, a feather fallen from a flying finch, or a gust of wind all become our reminders of unknown spirits. When we see the divine in someone's eyes, in someone's voice, in someone's sorrow, then we truly can see the sacred. God is the whisper between two friends.

When we live in our heart,
We celebrate the sacred.

According to the article, *Faith & Healing: Can prayer, faith and spirituality really improve your physical health?*, Herbert Benson, M.D., says that humans are biologically engineered for religious faith. "In a five-year study of patients using meditation to battle chronic illnesses,

Benson found that those who claim to feel the intimate presence of a higher power had better health and more rapid recoveries."[9]

A practical way of bringing the presence of a higher power into our lives is to celebrate the sacred. We can do this by bringing synchronicity, "coincidences," into every day and following its guidance. At the age of 16, Einstein had a synchronistic vision. In his daydreams, he used to ride a beam of light from the beginning to the end of creation. This set the stage for his lifelong search to mathematically explain the mysteries of the universe.

When I came to America, I experienced many synchronicities. For example, when I bought my first car in California, I scanned the entire classified section, and called only one person, because I was drawn to their ad. When I arrived at their home in Westwood, California the car's owners had participated in the same conference where I taught. The second coincidence was that although I had not met them physically they had heard of me. Since I am a believer of such meaningful coincidences, I bought my first car on Christmas Eve based completely on my intuition. I enjoyed this car for years, and it never gave me any problems.

This book was born in a castle on a hilltop over looking the panorama of the City of Angels. The first time I met Mickey Hargitay, the castle's builder and owner, he said, "I know you from two thousand years ago. I don't need to see any papers or sign anything. The place is yours. Here are the keys."

We all have coincidences in our lives. Do we ignore them as frivolous, or carefully listen to their message?

When we open our ears to coincidence,
We open our hearts to God.

All that is required is trust, and that can be challenging because it is tops on our list of don'ts. Like Nike, I say *just do it.*

Making altars is another way of celebrating the sacred in everyday living. We can build altars anywhere and everywhere. In our walk of life, we find many things which have special meaning for us, like a postcard from a friend, a feather from a bird, a fallen leaf from a tree, an idol or image given to us by a loved one. All can be used as sacred energies on our altars, reminders of Spirit energies we have attracted in this lifetime. The sacred is a window to spiritual power. In day to day life, by creating a quiet, poignant moment to go to our altar and offer our silence, our gratitude, or a candle, we energize Spirit. In the modem busy world I have found altars to be a place of solace. When we are hurt we can return to our altar. When we need to talk to someone we can speak in silence upon the altar. It is a divine couch given to us by spirit. We are invited to come and pour out our hearts.

Spirit of Prayer

Prayer is an essential rite of spirit. When two or more are connected, one can affect another in profound ways through the power of prayer. In my Healer's Journey, out of all my revelations, the one that has had the biggest effect in my self-healing is prayer. More than a decade has passed, and not a single day has gone where my mother has not sent her duaah (blessing vibrations) to me. Duaah is sending prayer energies with all of our consciousness. I am alive and completely well because of her duaah. Medicine can help, up to a point. When medicine fails, the only thing that works, as my experience indicates, is duaah.

When I was diagnosed with cancer, which had spread to many parts of my body, and I had no hope, what brought me back to life was duaah. I still remember that when I was being taken to the operating room on a gurney, everyone in my family, in London and in India, was at that time praying and sending duaah. When I clinically died, and was leaving my body, the duaah from many hearts brought me back.

In America, I was selling paintings for about a year to support myself. One day an old couple stopped by the store. Without knowing my story, they shared with me that the man had cancer for many years. The old woman said with confidence and grace, "Even though he has had cancer for many years nothing will happen to him because I don't believe it will. My husband will live a full life." I believed that her trust and faith changed his destiny. I believed in her. "My husband will live a full life" was her duaah.

> *Prayer is not a rehearsal.*
> *Prayer is a recital of Spirit.*

True wealth is not measured by the price of our possessions but by how much duaah we have in our lives. Every act of prayer directed to another is the creation of duaah. When we offer duaah to others, we receive blessings ourselves. The benefits are the same, whether giving or receiving; that is the beauty of Spirit. Duaah comes from the place of oneness with others.

How To Do Duaah

The only qualification for duaah is feeling oneness with the person with whom we are sharing. The way to feel the oneness is by empathy, not sympathy. Sympathy is extending security that, in return, makes the other person dependent on the sympathizer. Such molly-coddling makes both persons weak. In contrast, empathy is to be fully present with someone, listening to their feelings without attempting to minimize their discomfort or rescue them. We allow the other person to freely be themself without judging them or trying to change them. This empowers the other person. Transformation happens within this circle of understanding. For example, if someone we are dealing with is codependent or alcoholic, we do not criticize or sympathize. We instead feed them power by sincerely listening to them and offering duaah.

When we are offering duaah in another's presence, we can take the palm of our hand and by simple compassion we can touch them. Touch heals. When someone is at a distance awaiting our duaah, we hold an image of our long-distance dear one in our mind and heart. If we experience difficulties recreating this image, we can use a picture or letter to help bridge the distance, or we can simply send duaah by intuitive connectedness. It works as effectively long-distance as tete-a-tete.

THE HEALING POWER OF PRAYER

I always culminate my seminar by offering healing prayers to all as a gift. Spirit gave me my life back, and to celebrate Spirit I always offer healing prayers wherever I teach. Knowledge may change us but prayer will transform us, even if we are not consciously aware of it. The following is a true account of the power of prayer.

I am a registered nurse of 25 years experience, primarily with critically ill patients. In the fall of 1994 in San Diego, CA, I attended a healing prayer circle facilitated by Rahul Patel. There were approximately 200 people present. Rahul instructed the group to send out prayers to anyone we wanted, and the group did this while holding hands and hearing high vibrational sounds. The energy in the room was intense, and I was visualizing and sending prayer to my brother who lived in Chicago. It was approximately 4:30 in the afternoon, which was 6:30 in Chicago. The very next morning I called my mother in Chicago to find out haw my brother was doing and she sounded upset. I asked her what was going on. She told me that approximately 6:30 in the evening my brother was in a car with his friend, stopped in heavy traffic in downtown Chicago, when a group of men broke the windshield out on the car with baseball bats and beat my brother's friend unconscious. My brother managed to come out unharmed from this potentially fatal situation... I witnessed the miracle of the nonlocal Intelligence in the powerful prayer of Rahul Patel.   Sincerely, Beverly Hadley, R.N.[10]

My colleague and friend, Larry Dossey, M.D. illustrates the effect of prayer in *Healing Words: The Power of Prayer and the Practice of Medicine*. After a decade of research, Dr. Dossey summarized that the "empirical evidence for prayer's power is indirect evidence for the soul."[11] We can be inspired to include prayer in medicine. According to a Time/CNN poll, 82% of Americans believe in the healing power of prayer, and 64% think that doctors should pray with patients upon their request.[12]

HOLOGRAM OF HEALING

A **hologram** is a universal blueprint of the past, present and future all contained in an instant glimpse of the whole. It is the map we use to chart our desired destinies. The hologram is the ocean of possibilities and we are a drop from that same fathomless ocean. The key to opening our hologram is our conscious choice. The discovery of the hologram can only come by experience, by taking a leap of faith into the sea of uncertainty. Lao Tse said in *Tao Te Ching*, "The more you know, the less you understand." Our mind is the interference in understanding the hologram.

My quest for healing took me around the world. I saw the hologram of *The Healer's Way: An Inner Guide to Healing Through Energy Medicine* during my sojourn. My consciousness guided me to Susan in Sacramento where I was teaching at the Evolving Times Expo in 1998. Without knowing anything about her professional background, I entered the hologram. Susan, based on her own belief in the hologram, came to the City of Angels and made this her new home for three months. Every day, showers or shine, she was there with her laptop computer. When one is open, willingness and surrender enable us to manifest the potential of the hologram.

Everyone on earth is born with a unique, divine blueprint. We are all part of God. When we enter into our hologram by making conscious choices we become whole. Sufi mystic Indries Shah wrote *The Book of the Book*. Only sixteen pages have been written. The rest of the book consists of empty pages. We must take a journey of the soul to find the ocean. In doing that, we can fill the empty pages in *The Book of the Book* of our life.

How We Enter the Hologram

We enter the hologram when we reach a point of **critical mass**, as in high-energy physics where transmutation takes place when energy reaches critical mass. Nothing happens before this point of transition, no matter how hard or how much we try. Our will is the vehicle that takes us to that point. But we enter the hologram when we connect with Spirit by surrendering. Surrender is our lover aspect. The healer is born out of the interplay between the warrior and the lover, the synergy of will and surrender. It is then that we open our hologram.

No one ever flew before the Wright Brothers. Why? Because the Wright Brothers had enough will to keep trying in spite of uncountable failures. They also surrendered to their imagination, and did not succumb to public opinion. This simple synergy of will and surrender enabled them to enter the hologram of flying. It propelled them into the skies of their dreams.

When one person enters the hologram, it literally alters the vibrations in the energy field which, in turn, affects the whole universe. Brian Browne Walker says, in his translation of the *I Ching*, "In a very real sense the progress of the world depends upon your progress as an individual."¹³ This process spontaneously motivates others to go through the sound barrier-breaking through the barrier of the brain, the load of logic, the limitations of our minds based on past conditioning. There is a ripple effect that causes a shift in others' awareness, and more people enter the hologram. This phenomenon can be witnessed every four years in the Olympics. If someone can do it *why not me?*.

We go beyond.
We go for the gold.

Holographic healing affects all aspects of life. In the new millennium, cultural disease patterns will change as we experience a collective shift in consciousness and enter into a new hologram. I envision that cancer will not be as common, and will become a rare occurrence in the future. Life with AIDS will be helped by many alternative modalities, and we will not suffer from a scarcity of resources. The major illnesses of the past will be effectively healed, like tuberculosis and the common cold.

Spirit is the zenith of transformation. Spirit is energy, and that is why energy can heal. Nothing dies in the realm of energy or in the world of Spirit. When someone departs, the Spirit of that person does not die. Their vibrations remain in the etheric world. If we need their help, their guidance, their connection, their love, they will always come to us in silence whenever we simply acknowledge their presence. Nothing dies in God's world. It simply changes form. When a door shuts on us, somewhere else many new doors are opening in our hologram.

In *The Man Who Planted Trees*,¹⁴ the author tells a story of a man who enters a new hologram when his wife and child die. He begins planting 100 acorns every day. At the end of his life, he has transformed a barren valley into a forest of trees, a living symbol of celebration and hope. People come from all over the world to visit his Garden of Eden.

This story of how, when one door is slammed shut, another can open, has inspired readers for twenty-five years.

THE LAW OF OPPOSITES

Life is a paradox. We are often caught in dichotomy. One day we love someone, another day we think we hate the same person. One day we create with our hearts, the next we destroy with our minds. Nothing is good, and nothing is bad. Both are parts of the same play. The first time we try to swim we sink. When we float effortlessly, we continue in the flow. When we try to win we lose. The secret of life is to be, action without action. In our most trying times, the more extreme our conditions are, the more chances we have to overcome them. We can turn our dilemmas into advantages if we do not give up.

Carl Hammerschlag, M.D. was treating a Pueblo priest named Santiago.[15] Santiago inquired about Dr. Hammerschlag's background in healing. Trained as a psychiatrist at Yale University, he produced a dossier of professional qualifications. The old priest then asked, "Do you know how to dance? You must be able to dance if you are to heal people... I can teach you my steps, but you will have to hear your own music."

When we find our song we find ourselves. The journey of a healer is the journey of the eternal hero. By reliving our pain, we relieve it. When we share the very thing we desire, we heal ourselves. It is not the golden chalice that counts, it is the journey of the chalice that matters in the realm of Spirit.

I was lost. I was looking for my home. Where could I find it? I was like a drop leaving the known cloud, going into the unknown. Splash!! While doing my healing work, when I looked in your eyes, when I looked in your hearts, I found oneness. In this oneness, I found my home.

God is energy. We all have a divine song, our unique talent. By singing our song we live with God. We are all a pirouette of possibilities. It is about love. Love heals. Love heals all paradoxes.

The more we give,
The more we create transformation.

We have met many lifetimes before, although we may have not met physically, and we will meet again and again…

EXERCISES FOR TRANSFORMATION AND HEALING

1. **Do What We Like, Like What We Do:** Take an instant inventory of things in our lives that bring us joy and fulfillment. Find five things that we love to do. Then let go of five shoulds. Job satisfaction deeply affects our health and happiness. Write a description of our dream job. This plants the seed to manifest the job we want. Water it with positive intentions.

2. **Attracting Abundance:** Each time we bring new energies into our lives that enrich us, we change our patterns. For example, we can bring new supportive friends, new affirmations, or keep a journal of our blessings. Write a wish list of the things we want to attract in our lives. Read this list at least once in the morning and evening each day for three months, and continue with gentle persistence. Be prepared to receive Santas, even in summer!

3. **Celebrate Spirit:** Light a candle, make an altar and create a sacred space in our usual environment. Begin the day by visiting our altar. It is a great place to keep our wish lists! Choose an inspirational saying that becomes our offering to spirit.

NOTES

1. It is illustrated in the book *Akashic Records: Past Lives and New Directions* by Robert Chaney.

2. See Lee Coit's fine book *Listening: How to Increase Awareness of Your Inner Guide* for techniques to help us recognize these messages.

3. George Gurdjieff, the modern mystic, describes this in his book, *All and Everything*.

4. City University of New York, New York.

5. *Much Ado about Nothing*, Act II, Scene I, Line 351, William Shakespeare.

6. See Richard Bach's *The Bridge Across Forever*.

7. Harvard researcher Herbert Benson, M.D., has documented gtummo in film.

8. *The Essential Rumi* translated by Coleman Barks with John Moyne, p. 185.

9. *Time*, June 24, 1996, p. 61.

10. This letter was dated December 27, 1998 with full authorization for its use by Beverly Hadley.

11. *The Power of Prayer and the Practice of Medicine* by Larry Dossey, M.D., back cover.

12. *Time*, June 24, 1996.

13. The *I Ching: A Guide to Life's Turning Points* by Brian Browne Walker, p. 93.

14. *The Man Who Planted Trees*, by Jean Giorno.

15. From the back cover of *The Dancing Healers: A Doctor's Journey of Healing with Native Americans.*

TERMAS

Prescription For Happiness

Termas is an ancient tradition in Tibetan Buddhism. In my Tibetan trek I participated first-hand in healing techniques, and learned about the word **termas**, hidden treasures and teachings. Termas are revealed to a suitable person at the appropriate time.

I believe termas are the messages of daily enlightenment that we attract through our awareness. When we are divinely guided by strangers or receive a message unexpectedly, all of these have the potential to enhance our life force. We often miss these messages because we do not pay attention to them, or if we do, we tend to dismiss them as insignificant. By listening we can attract messages that help guide our steps and enables our hidden potential to unfold. In the world of energy, everything is vibration. By attracting enriching vibrations we can create our new destiny.

How do we attract termas? Here is an interesting example. When I was copying the manuscript of this book I attracted a stranger who gravitated toward the different piles of chapters I was arranging. He scanned through all of the piles. He came to me and said, "Everything in the universe has a spirit. If you feel the vibrations, then you are connected."

This strange man delivered my termas from Spirit. My awareness attracted this messenger to remind me of energy, the interconnectedness with Spirit, the essence of *The Healer's Way: An Inner Guide to Healing Through Energy Medicine*. "If you feel the vibrations, then you are connected."

Termas, messages of our happiness, are all around us. We need to start listening and paying attention to them. Life is not *to be or not to be?* **Life is all and everything.**

Life is not a compromise. We must take a leap into the unknown in order to unfold our hologram. The prescription of happiness requires being willing to take risks to uncover the special talent with which we are born – living our dharma – and celebrating it as a cherished gift with a burning hope.

Siddhartha, the eternal seeker, is searching for his termas to discover his dharma, the purpose and meaning of his life. He goes through an odyssey that takes him from courtesan to sanyasi (a renunciate). Evolving from sensual pleasures to spiritual bliss, Siddhartha finds his dharma on the banks of the river. He realizes that the flow of the river is the essence of life. "Is it you, Siddhartha? I can see in your eyes that you have found enlightenment," Govinda said.[1] Siddhartha paused, plucked a stone, and put it in his hand, saying, "This stone is a stone, it is also an animal, it is also God, it is also the Buddha, I love and honor it not because it could become this or that someday, but because it is everything long since and always…"[2]

Life is a journey of flow. In my journey, knowingly or unknowingly, if I have hurt anyone, I ask for forgiveness…

NOTES

1. Paraphrased by the author.
2. Nobel laureate Hermann Hesse's *Siddhartha*, p. 126.

❧

ACKNOWLEDGMENTS

Gratitude to Extraordinary People

Though there are as many angels who have helped me in my life as there are stars in the sky, space only permits me to acknowledge these few:

My father & mother: For your constant duaah and prayers that gave me energy to live and love life. Without you, I would not have been able to give birth to this book.

Milton Katselas: For sharing your friendship, the power of abundance and innumerable generosities with me.

Bernie Siegel: For teaching the medicine of love that created the healing miracle for me when I needed it most.

Louise Hay: For helping me to let go of the past and showing me how to live fully by loving my inner child.

Deepak Chopra: For sharing and celebrating the Spirit which gave me a reason to live. It elevated my ordinary into extraordinary.

Neale Donald Walsch: For your gracious vision, your giant heart, your *Conversations with God* and your support.

Larry Dossey: For opening your heart with compassion that evoked the power of prayer in my daily life.

Kathy Smith & Russell Kamalski: For your belief, support and kindness, which were instrumental to this book.

Mickey Hargitay: Whose soul, friendship and faith in me have helped me in difficult times and throughout this book.

George Solomon: For sharing psychoneuro-immunology and many sessions where you inspired me to health.

Brendan O'Regan & Caryle Hirshberg: Whose research helped me to know that spontaneous remission is a reality.

Cleve Backster: The genius who demonstrated that I can "talk" to my removed cells effectively, even at a distance.

Susan Saccaro: My primary editorial assistant whose simple dedication and clarity are unsurpassable. I admire you.

Dennis Rodgers: Whose editorial assistance and insights helped me to complete this book. I value your friendship.

Helena Stockwell: For your constant communication, friendship and belief in me, which inspired me in the journey of this book.

Carol Stumphauzer: Your friendship inspired me to grow in many ways; for your belief and support I am grateful.

Nancy Kahan: Whose understanding, support insight and dedication have opened new frontiers.

Sandy Sumich: Whose heart-felt energy and guidance gave me feedback and support to complete the book.

Stacy Meyn: For your constant guidance and insight that grew into this book.

Richard Launey: For tireless contribution of your computer expertise and immediate response to SOS calls.

Kerry Slattery: For your editorial support and sharing your valuable experience that helped me with the book.

Ken Babal: For sharing your nutritional expertise and suggestions for the book.

Baldev Bhai: For your friendship, support and ongoing insights.

Jay Gilbert: For your trust and gracious friendship that remain with me always.

Meher Amalsad: For sharing your "bread for the head" wisdom with me.

James Ha: For your friendship and constant belief in me.

❖

REFERENCES

A Wider Hearing. Psillos, D. *Vogue (British)*, June, 1992, p. 169-170.

Ackerman, D. *A Natural History of the Senses.* New York: Vintage Books, 1990.

Awana, R. *Radiation: The Hidden Enemy.* Lawrenceville, NJ: Princeton Academic Press Inc., 1994.

Bach, R. *The Bridge Across Forever: A love story.* New York: Dell Publishing, 1984.

Bachler, Kathe. *Earth Radiation: The Startling Discoveries of a Dowser: Results of Research on more than 3,000 apartments, houses, and work places.* Mancester, England: Wordmasters Ltd., 1976.

Baker, I. *The Tibetan Art of Healing.* San Francisco: Chronicle Books, 1997.

Beaulieu, J. *Music and Sound in the Healing Arts: An Energy Approach.* Barrytown, NY: Station Hill Press, 1987.

Becker, R. *Cross Currents: The Promise of Electromedicine, The Perils of Electropollution.* Los Angeles: Jeremy P. Tarcher, Inc., 1990.

Benson, H. with Stark, M. *Timeless Healing: The Power and Biology of Belief.* New York: Scribner, 1996.

Besserman, P. & Steger, M. *Crazy Clouds: Zen Radicals, Rebels & Reformers.* Boston: Shambhala, 1991.

Bird, C. *The Divining Hand: The art of searching for water, oil, minerals, and other natural resources or anything lost, missing or badly needed.* Black Mountain, NC: New Age Press, 1979.

Black Elk, W. and Lyon, W. *Black Elk: The Sacred Ways of A Lakota.* New York: HarperCollins Publishers, 1990.

Bourre, J. *Brainfood: A Provocative Exploration of the Connection Between What You Eat and How You Think.* Boston: Little, Brown and Company, 1993.

Bruyere, R. *Wheels of Light : Chakras, Auras, and the Healing Energy of the Body.* New York: Simon & Schuster, 1989.

Cancer and Diet. Cowley, G. *Newsweek,* November 30, 1998, p.60-66.

Cancer: Do We Already Have a "Cure"? Walters, R. *Body Mind & Spirit,* January/February, 1991, p. 40-45.

Carper, J. *Food – Your Miracle Medicine: How Food Can Prevent and Cure Over 100 Symptoms and Problems.* New York: HarperPerennial, 1993.

Chopra, D. *Ageless Body, Timeless Mind: The Quantum Alternative to Growing Old.* New York: Harmony Books, 1993.

Chuen, L. *Feng Shui Handbook: How to Create a Healthy Living and Working Environment.* New York: Henry Holt and Company, 1996.

Coghill, R. *Electro Pollution: How to protect yourself against it.* Northamptonshire, England: Thorsons Publishing Group, 1990.

Cohen, K. *The Way of Qigong: The Art and the Science of Chinese Energy Healing.* New York: Ballantine Books, 1997.

Colbin, A. *Food and Healing.* New York: Ballantine Books, 1986.

Collinge, W. *Subtle Energy: Awakening to the Unseen Forces in Our Lives.* New York: Warner Books, 1998.

Conservation, Ethnobotany, and the Search for New Jungle Medicines: Pharmacognosy Comes of Age Again. Plotkin, M. *Pharmacotherapy,* Vol. 8, No. 5, 1988, p. 257-262.

Cowan, D. and Girdlestone, R. *Safe As Houses?: Ill Health and Electro-stress in the Home.* Bath, UK: Gateway Books, 1995.

Davies, R. *Dowsing: Ancient origins and modern uses.* Hammersmith, London: The Aquarian Press, 1991.

Day, C. *Places of the Soul: Architecture and Environmental Design as a Healing Art.* San Francisco: Aquarian/Thorsons, 1990.

Dossey, L. *Healing Words: The Power of Prayer and The Practice of Medicine.* New York: HarperCollins Publishers, 1993.

Dossey, L. *Meaning & Medicine: Lessons from a Doctor's Tales of Breakthrough and Healing.* New York: Bantam Books, 1991.

Dossey, L. *Prayer is Good Medicine: How to Reap the Healing Benefits of Prayer.* New York: HarperCollins Publishers, 1996.

Dossey, L. *Recovering the Soul: A Scientific and Spiritual Search.*New York: Bantam Books, 1989.

Dowman, K. (translator). *The Divine Madman: The Sublime Life and Songs of Drukpa Kunley.* Middletown, CA: The Dawn Horse Press, 1980.

Dychtwald, K. *Body-Mind.* New York: Pantheon Books, 1977.

Eaton, S., Shostak, M., and Kanner, M. *The Paleolithic Prescription: A Program of Diet & Exercise and A Design for Livrng.* New York: Harper & Row, Publishers, 1988.

Effects of Harmful Radiations and Noxious Rays: A Series of Research Papers by Noted Scientists and Authors, Danville, VT: American Society of Dowsers, Inc., 1974.

ElectroMagnetic Fields: In Search of the Truth. Cunningham, A. *Popular Science,* December, 1991, p. 87-91.

Elkort, M. *The Secret Life of Food: A Feast of Food and Drink History, Folklore and Fact.* Los Angeles: Jeremy P. Tarcher, 1991.

Faith and Healing: Can prayer, faith and spirituality really improve your physical health? Wallis, C. *Time,* June 24, 1996, p. 59-68.

Fincher, S. *Creating Mandalas: For Insight, Healing, and Self Expression*. Boston: Shambhala, 1991.

Firshein, R. *The Nutraceutical Revolution: 20 Cutting-Edge Nutrients to Help You Design Your Own Perfect Whole-life Program*. New York: Riverhead Books, 1998.

Ford, C. *Compassionate Touch: The Role of Human Touch in Healing and Recovery*. New York: A Fireside/Parkside Book, 1993.

Frankl, V. *Man's Search for Meaning: An Introduction to Logotherapy*. New York: Pocket Books, 1959.

Gallagher, W. *The Power of Place: How Our Surroundings Shape Our Thoughts, Emotions, and Actions*. New York: Poseidon Press, 1993.

Geller, U. and Playfair, G. *The Geller Effect*. New York: Henry Holt and Company, 1986.

Georgakas, D. *The Methuselah Factors: Learning From the World's Longest Living People*. Chicago: Academy Chicago Publishers, 1995.

Gilmor, T., Madaule, P. and Thompson, B. *About the Tomatis Method*. Toronto: Tomatis, 1989.

Gleick, J. *Chaos: Making a New Science*. New York: Penguin Books, 1987.

Godwin, M. *Angels: An Endangered Species*. New York: Simon and Schuster, 1990.

Goldman, J. *Healing Sounds: The Power of Harmonics*. Shaftesbury, Dorset: Element, 1992.

Goleman, D. and Gurin, J. (eds.). *MindBody Medicine: How To Use Your Mind For Better Health*. Yonkers, NY: Consumer Reports Books, 1993.

Gottman, J. *Why Marriages Succeed or Fail... and How You Can Make Yours Last.* New York: Simon &. Schuster, 1994.

Groves, D. *Feng-Shui and Western Building Ceremonies.* Singapore: Graham Brash, 1991.

Guiley, R. *The Miracle of Prayer: True Stories of Blessed Healings.* New York: Pocket Books, 1995.

Hageseth Ill, C. *A Laughing Place: The Art and Psychology of Positive Humor in Love and Adversity.* Fort Collins, CO: Berwick Publishing Company, 1988.

Hammerschlag, C. *The Dancing Healers: A Doctor's Journey of Healing with Native Americans.* New York: HarperCollins Publishers, 1988.

Hay, L. *You Can Heal Your Life.* Carson, CA: Hay House, Inc., 1984.

Hirshberg, C. & Barasch, M. *Remarkable Recovery: What Extraordinary Healings Tell Us About Getting Well and Staying Well.* New York: Riverhead Books, 1995.

Hover-Kramer, D. *Healing Touch: A Resource for Health Care Professionals.* Albany, NY: Delmar Publishers, 1996.

Hutchison, M. *Mega Brain Power: Transform Your Life With Mind Machines and Brain Nutrients.* New York: Hyperion, 1994.

Iovine, J. *Kirlian Photography: A Hands-On Guide.* Blue Ridge Summit, PA: TAB Books, 1994.

Katselas, M. *Dreams Into Action: Getting What You Want!* Beverly Hills, CA: Dove Books, 1996.

Keller, D. *Humor as Therapy.* Wauwatosa, WI: Med-Psych Publications, 1984.

Kingston, J. *Healing Without Medicine*. London: The Danbury Press, 1975.

Klein, A. *The Healing Power of Humor: Techniques for Getting through Loss, Setbacks, Upsets, Disappointments, Difficulties, Trials, Tribulations, and All That Not-So-Funny Stuff*. New York: Jeremy P. Tarcher/Putnam,1989.

Krieger, D. *The Personal Practice of Therapeutic Touch: Accepting Your Power to Heal*. Santa Fe, NM: Bear & Company Publishing, 1993.

Krieger, D. *The Therapeutic Touch: How to Use Your Hands to Help or to Heal*. New York: Prentice Hall Press, 1979.

Krippner, S. and Villoldo, A. *The Realms of Healing* (New Revised Edition). Millbrae, CA: Celestial Arts, 1976.

Kushi, M. *The Book of Macrobiotics: The Universal Way of Health and Happiness*. Toyko: Japan Publications, Inc., 1977.

Lakhovsky, G. *The Secret of Life: Cosmic Rays and Radiations of Living Beings*. Martino Fine Books. 2013.

Langer, E. *Mindfulness*. Reading, MA: Addison-Wesley Publishing Company, Inc., 1989.

Le Guerer, A. *Scent: The Mysterious and Essential Powers of Smell*. New York: Turtle Bay Books, 1992.

Levitt, B. *Electromagnetic Fields: A Consumer's Guide to the Issues and How to Protect Ourselves*. San Diego: Harcourt Brace & Company, 1995.

Liberman, J. *Light: Medicine of the Future: How We Can Use It to Heal Ourselves NOW*. Santa Fe, N.M.: Bear & Company Publishing, 1991.

Lillian Too's Basic Feng Shui: An Illustrated reference manual (North American Edition). Adelaide, South Australia: Oriental Publications, 1997.

Lip, E. *Feng Shui for the home*. Singapore: Heian International, Inc., 1990.

Lipp, F. *Herbalism, Healing and Harmony: Symbolism, Ritual, and Folklore Traditions of East and West*. Boston: Little, Brown and Company, 1996.

Locke, S. and Colligan, D. *The Healer Within: The New Medicine of Mind and Body*. New York: New American Library, 1986.

Macrae, J. *Therapeutic Touch: A Practical Guide*. New York: Alfred A. Knopf, 1987.

Magic and Medicine of Plants. Pleasantville, NY: The Reader's Digest Association, Inc., 1986.

Majno, G. *The Healing Hand: Man and Wound in the Ancient World*. Cambridge, MA: Harvard University Press, 1975.

Masson, J. and McCarthy, S. *When Elephants Weep: The Emotional Lives of Animals*. New York: Delacorte Press, 1995.

McAleer, N. *The Body Almanac: Mind-Boggling Facts About Today's Human Body and High-Tech Medicine*. New York: Doubleday & Company, Inc., 1985.

McClellan, R. *The Healing Forces of Music: History, Theory & Practice*. Rockport, MA: Element, 1991.

McGee, C., and Chow, E. *Miracle Healing from China: Qigong*. Coeur d'Alene, ID: MediPress, 1994.

McGhee, P. *Health, Healing and the Amuse System: Humor as Survival Training* (Second Edition). Dubuque, IA: Kendall/Hunt Publishing Company, 1996.

McGhee, P. *The Laughter Remedy: Health, Healing, and the Amuse System*. Montclair, N.J.: Paul McGhee, 1991.

Milburn, M. and Oelbermann, M. *Electromagnetic Fields and Your Health: What You Need to Know About the Hidden Hazards of Electricity – and How You Can Protect Yourself.* Vancouver: New Star Books, 1994.

Montagu, A. *Growing Young.* New York: Bergin & Garvey Publishers, 1981.

Moss, T. *The Probability of the Impossible: Scientific Discoveries and Explorations in the Psychic World.* Los Angeles: J.P. Tarcher, Inc., 1974.

Moyers, B. *Healing and the Mind.* New York: Doubleday, 1993.

Mr. Natural. Kluger, J. *Time,* May 12, 1997, p. 68-75.

Myers, D. *The Pursuit of Happiness: Who is Happy – and Why.* New York: William Morrow and Company, Inc., 1992.

Myss, C. *Why People Don't Heal and How They Can.* New York: Harmony Books, 1997.

Natale, F. *Trance Dance: The Dance of Life.* Shaftesbury, Dorset: Element, 1995.

Nature's Healing Arts: From Folk Medicine to Modern Drugs. Washington DC: National Geographic Society, 1977.

Neuroendocrine and Stress Hormone Changes During Mirthful Laughter. Berk, L., Tan, S. and Fry, W. et al. *The American Journal of The Medical Sciences,* December, 1989, p. 390-96.

O'Regan, B. and Hirshberg, C. *Spontaneous Remission: An Annotated Bibliography.* Sausalito, CA: Institute of Noetic Sciences, 1993.

Oldfield, H. and Coghill, R. *The Dark Side of the Brain: Major Discoveries in the Use of Kirlian Photography and Electrocrystal Therapy.* Shaftesbury, Dorset: Element Books, 1988.

On The Road Again. Woodward, K. *Newsweek,* November 28, 1994, p. 53-62.

Ornish, D. *Dr. Dean Ornish's Program for Reversing Heart Disease: The Only System Scientifically Proven to Reverse Heart Disease Without Drugs or Surgery.* New York: Ballantine Books, 1990.

Ornish, D. *Love and Survival: The Scientific Basis for the Healing Power of Intimacy.* New York: HarperCollins Publishers, 1997.

Ornstein, R. and Sobel, D. *Healthy Pleasures.* Reading, MA: Addison-Wesley Publishing Company, Inc., 1989.

Ornstein, R. and Swencionis, C. (eds.). *The Healing Brain: A Scientific Reader.* New York: Guilford Press, 1990.

Panic over Power Lines: Are the Waves From Electrical Wires and Appliances Harmful? Toufexis, A. *Time,* July 17, 1989, p. 71.

Patnaik, N. *The Garden of Life: An Introduction To The Healing Plants of India.* New York: Doubleday, 1993.

Payer, L. *Medicine and Culture: Varieties of Treatment in the United States, England, West Germany, and France.* New York: Penguin Books, 1988.

Pennick, N. *Earth Harmony: Siting and Protecting Your Home – a Practical and Spiritual Guide.* London: Century, 1987.

Perry, S. and Dawson, J. *The Secrets Our Body Clocks Reveal.* New York: Rawson Associates, 1988.

Pinsky, M. *The EMF Book: What You Should Know About Electromagnetic Fields, Electromagnetic Radiation, and Your Health.* New York: Warner Books, 1995.

Plotkin, M. *Tales of a Shaman's Apprentice: An Ethnobotanist Searches for New Medicines in the Amazon Rain Forest.* New York: Viking, 1993.

Potter, B. and Orfali, S. *Brain Boosters: Foods & Drugs that Make You Smarter.* Berkeley, CA: Ronin Publishing, Inc., 1993.

Radin, D. *The Conscious Universe: The Scientific Truth of Psychic Phenomena.* San Francisco: HarperEdge, 1997.

Random-number psi effect valid, review concludes. Los Angeles: *Brain/ Mind Bulletin*, April 1990, Vol. 15, No. 7, p. 1-2.

Reid, D. *Harnessing the Power of the Universe: A Complete Guide to the Principles and Practice of Chi-Gung.* Boston: Shambhala, 1998.

Rinpoche, T. *Hidden Teachings of Tibet: An Explanation of the Terma Tradition of Tibetan Buddhism.* Boston: Wisdom Publications, 1986.

Roney-Dougal, S. *Where Science & Magic Meet.* Shaftesbury, Dorset: Element, 1991.

Root-Bernstein , R. and Root-Bernstein, M. *Honey, Mud, Maggots, and Other Medical Marvels: The Science Behind Folk Remedies and Old Wives' Tales.* Boston: Houghton Mifflin Company, 1997.

Rossbach, S. *Interior Design with Feng Shui.* New York: Arkana, 1987.

Rossbach, S. and Yun, L. *Living Color: Master Lin Yun's Guide to Feng Shui and the Art of Color.* New York: Kodansha. International, 1994.

Sargent, D. *Global Ritualism: Myth & Magic Around The World.* St. Paul, MN: Llewellyn Publications, 1994.

Schechter, S. *Fighting Radiation with Foods, Herbs, & Vitamins: Documented Natural Remedies that Protect You from Radiation, X-Rays, & Chemical Pollutants.* Brookline, MA: East West Health Books, 1988.

Schul, B. *Life Song: In Harmony with All Creation.* Walpole, NH: Stillpoint Publishing, 1994.

Scientific Investigations into Chinese Qi-Gong. San Clemente, CA: China Healthways Institute, 1992.

Seligman, M. *Learned Optimism: How to Change Your Mind and Your Life.* New York: Pocket Books , 1990.

Shah, I. *The Book of the Book* in *The Indries Shah Anthology.* London: The ISF Foundation, 2019.

Shealy, C. *Miracles Do Happen: A Physician's Experience With Alternative Medicine.* Rockport, MA: Element, 1995.

Simonton, O. and Henson, R. *The Healing Journey.* New York: Bantam Books, 1992.

Snellgrove, B. *The Unseen Self: Kirlian Photography Explained.* Essex, England: The C.W. Daniel Company Limited, 1996.

Sobel, D. and Ornstein, R. *The Healthy Mind Healthy Body Handbook.* New York: Patient Education Media, Inc., 1996.

Spear, W. *Feng Shui Made Easy: Designing Your Life with the Ancient Art of Placement.* New York: HarperCollins Publishers, 1995.

Spintge, R. and Droh, R. (eds .). *Music Medicine.* St. Louis, MO: MMB Music, Inc., 1992.

Sternfield, J. *Firewalk: The Psychology of Physical Immunity.* Stockbridge, MA: Berkshire House Publishers, 1992.

Sugarman, E. *Warning: The Electricity Around You May Be Hazardous to Your Health: How to Protect Yourself from Electromagnetic Fields.* New York: Simon & Schuster, 1992.

Swan, J. *Nature as Teacher and Healer: How to Reawaken Your Connection with Nature.* New York: Villard Books, 1992.

Swartwout, G. *Electromagnetic Pollution Solutions: What You Can Do To Keep Your Home & Workplace Safe.* Hilo, Hawaii: Aerai Publishing, 1991.

Temoshok, L. and Dreher, H. *The Type C Connection: The Behavioral Links to Cancer and Your Health.* New York: Random House, 1992.

The health dangers of sleeping on a Hartmann line. Biser, S. *Health Discoveries Newsletter,* Issue #25, p. 1-3.

The Heart of Healing. The Institute of Noetic Sciences with William Poole. Atlanta: Turner Publishing, Inc., 1993.

The Nectar of Gaia. Steele, J. *Perfumer & Flavorist,* Vol. 15, July/ August 1990, p. 19-22.

Thumell-Read, J. *Geopathic Stress: How Earth Energies Affect Our Lives.* Shaftesbury, Dorset: Element, 1995.

Tsung, P. *Immune System and Chinese Herbs.* Irvine, CA: Institute of Chinese Herb, 1989.

Venolia, C. *Healing Environments: Your Guide to Indoor WellBeing.* Berkeley, CA: Celestial Arts, 1988.

Vitebsky, P. *The Shaman: Voyages of the Soul Trance, Ecstasy, and Healing from Siberia to the Amazon.* Boston: Little, Brown and Company, 1995.

Von Pohl, G. *Earth Currents: Causative Factor of Cancer and other Diseases.* Stuttgart, Germany: Frech-Verlag, 1978.

Waal, M. *Medicines from the Bible: Roots & Herbs & Woods & Oils.* York Beach, ME: Samuel Weiser, Inc., 1994.

Walsch, N. *Conversations with God: An Uncommon Dialogue, Book 3.* Charlottesville, VA: Hampton Roads Publishing Company, Inc., 1998.

Walsh, A. *The Science of Love: Understanding Love & Its Effects on Mind & Body.* Buffalo, NY: Prometheus Books, 1991.

Weil, A. *Spontaneous Healing: How to Discover and Enhance Your Body's Natural Ability to Maintain and Heal Itself.* New York: Alfred A. Knopf, 1995.

Why New Age Medicine Is Catching On. Wallis, C. *Time*, November 4, 1991, p. 68-76.

Wigmore, A. *The Wheatgrass Book.* Wayne , N.J.: Avery Publishing Group Inc., 1985 .

Wilson, C. *The Outsider.* Cambridge: The Riverside Press, 1956.

Winter , R. *A Consumer's Guide to Medicines in Food: Nutraceuticals That Help Prevent and Treat Physical and Emotional Illnesses.* New York: Crown Trade Paperbacks, 1995.

Wooten, P. *Compassionate Laughter: Jest for Your Health.* Salt Lake City, UT: Commune-A- Key Publishing, 1996.

Worwood, V. *The Complete Book of Essential Oils & Aromatherapy.* San Rafael, CA: New World Library, 1991.

INDEX

J

Jeffrey, Masson, Ph.D. 163
Jesus
  and the little children 129
  faith 8
  miracle of loaves and fishes 66
Juicing 69
Jung, Carl 146

K

Kabbala vii
Kahuna healers 37
kalavati 97
Katselas, Milton 14–15
Katz, Lawrence 95
Katz, Richard 27
ki 27
King, Dr. Stanley 48
Kipling, Rudyard 170
Kirlian photography 36, 70
Klein, Allen 133, 143
Kobasa, Suzanne, Ph.D. 168
Krutch, Joseph 156
Kübler-Ross, Dr. Elisabeth 14
kundalini 27
Kunley, Drukpa 140
Kushi, Michio 22

L

Lakhovsky, Georges 113, 123
Lancet, The 51
Langer, Ellen, Ph.D. 50
Lao Tse 21, 177
Laughing Buddha 129
laughter as healer 127–141
Law of Opposites 180
LeShan, Lawrence, Ph.D. 62, 163
life force 26–27
Light 11
lignans 71
Lily, John C., Ph.D. 93

listening 89, 182
  three phases of 90
Locke, Steven, M.D. 45
Longfellow, Henry Wadsworth 114
Lourdes 53
L-shaped rods 15
lung cancer 3
lycopene 72
lymphatic massage 68

M

macrobiotic approach 72, 85
magic 33, 120, 165
magical passes 13
Mahakasyapa 141
Maje me heh? 139
Majno, Guido, M.D. 26
malkauns (raga) 97
mandala 6, 21
Manners, Sir Peter Guy, M.D., Ph.D. 92
mantras 102–103
Maslow, Abraham 152
McClelland, David, Ph.D. 47, 56, 62
McGee, Paul, Ph.D. 132, 136, 143
medical school education 34
Meecham, William 93
metamorphosis 19
microelectric potential 70
microwave ovens 115
mindbody 45
Mind-Made Medicine 34
Mira Bai 130
miracle bag 162
miracle healing 148
miso soup 73
mistral 113
Monroe Institute, The 95
Montagu, Ashley 129
Moss, Thelma, Ph.D. 36
Mother Teresa Effect 56
music
  for crying infants 96

www.ingramcontent.com/pod-product-compliance
Lightning Source LLC
Chambersburg PA
CBHW031155270326
41931CB00006B/278